Reclaim Natural Beauty

*How to Grow, Nourish, and Strengthen
your Natural, Black Hair*

*****

This book is dedicated to all the beautiful black girls and women out there still searching to find themselves, and the inner fabulous that lives within them.

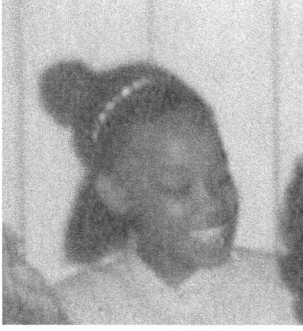
Me as a Child

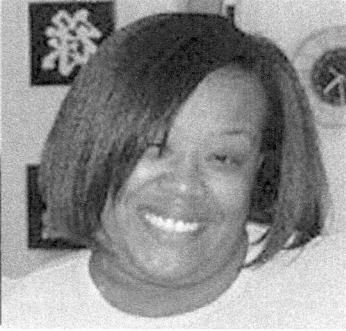
Before, with a Perm

BC after 6-Mnth transition
Feb, Yr 1

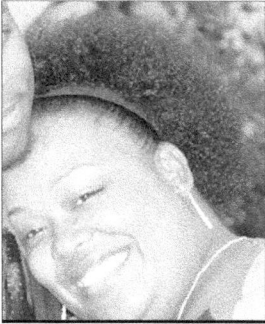
Afro – May, Yr 1

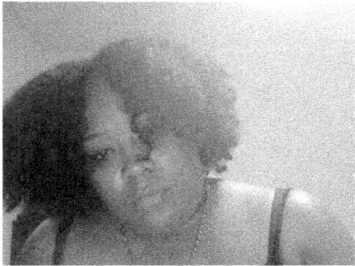
Twist-Outs – Jan, Yr 2

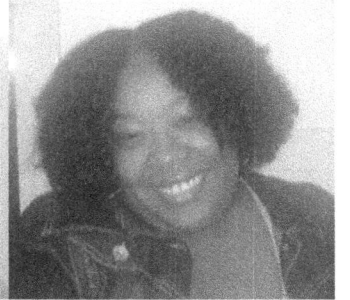
Braid-Outs – April, Yr 2

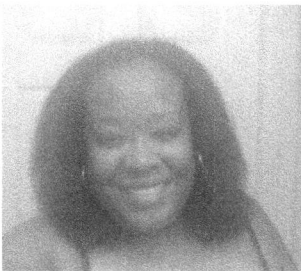
Flat Iron – April, Yr 2

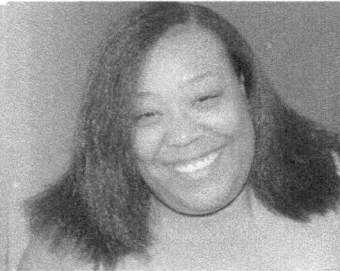
Flat-Iron – July, Yr 2

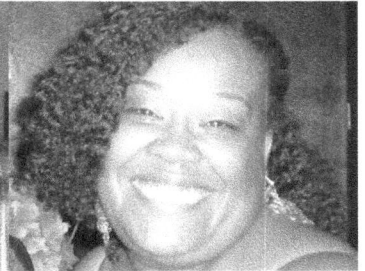
Twist-Outs – Aug, Yr. 2

Flat-Iron – Nov, Yr 2

Twist-Outs – Dec, Yr 2

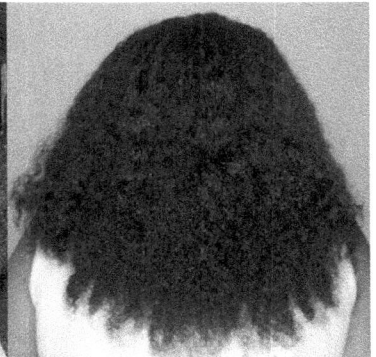
Total Span – 1 Yr, 10 Mnths

Table of Contents

Introduction | 1 |

Section 2: The Endless Possibilities with Natural Hair

Introduction

In recent times, there are so many women of color taking the world by storm with their beautiful, natural hair that it makes my heart swell with pride. More and more, you can see women everywhere you look with natural 'fros, curls, twists, braids, and dreadlocks. Despite this, however, there are still a great amount of women who have thought about going natural or may have even attempted it in the past, but were lacking information and really didn't know where to even begin; which made them either frustrated after a few months or afraid to go natural at all. Then there are other concerns: How they will be received, how to care for it, their options for styling, among others. When I first started this book, it was because I realized from my own experience how needed it was. When I decided to go natural, I was truly lost. I was frustrated, impatient, confused, and discouraged. I turned to the internet for information, and found myself flooded and lost amidst a sea of conflicting information, opinions, and rantings.

Though I feel differently now, when I first went natural, it was not with the intention of reclaiming any beauty at all. I didn't even know the "beauty" existed, I actually thought I was losing something. I had the same view of natural hair that many black women do, which oftentimes is, unfortunately, not very positive. The only thing I did know was that I was tired and fed up of one thing: the chemical relaxers. For several years, my hair was breaking and wouldn't stop. It was damaged from years of abuse and had no elasticity, and it would often snap and break off. I took the route of getting weaker perms, going to beauticians, cutting it, braiding it; I even went to a dermatologist. No matter what I did, certain sections of my hair would just not grow back properly. It never occurred to me in all the years I was having problems to actually stop relaxing my hair. Then one day, I just got tired and decided I was done. If I wanted my hair straight, then I would just straighten it with heat, but I wasn't relaxing it anymore. I believed that people would have a lot to say and not approve of my decision, but I just didn't care because I couldn't deal with the breakage anymore. The first several months were HELL (laugh), because I refused to just cut all my hair off and start over, so I was transitioning, and didn't really know how to do that either (we'll get more into that later). But after many months, I finally did my Big Chop, and the change in the state of my hair was like night and day. Then the reality quickly hit me: What now? I made the decision, but I really had no idea how to care for my new tresses. So I began to read. And read. And read some more. And the more I learned and implemented my newfound knowledge, the more I began to see positive changes in my hair that I never even knew could exist. Then, something else happened: Gradually, my decision to go natural became so much more than not using a relaxer because of breakage. Instead of wearing my natural hair despite the way it looked, I began to wear my hair natural because I *preferred* it that way. This change then grew into a feeling that I would never perm my hair again. I think it's a huge decision emotionally, as well as physically, when you learn to embrace your natural hair. I want others to feel the same way I do now about my hair, with a sense of pride in how beautiful their natural hair is or definitely can be. Every single woman I know that gets encouraged enough to make the change comes back to me and says things like, "I had no idea my hair could feel like that!" Or look like that, or grow that long; the revelations go on and on. It feels so good to see black women discover their natural hair and love it the way they do, which is usually such a big turnaround from the way they felt before. Even though it turns out to be as beautiful as I was telling them it would be, they really don't believe it until they're able to see and feel it for themselves.

Unlike what's been inbred in many of us from a young age, our hair is not ugly. It's not bad hair, it's not unruly, it's not unsightly, and it's not hard to the touch. If properly taken cared of, our hair is soft, manageable, can grow as long as other cultures, and is absolutely beautiful. To think that I had to become a grown woman before I could see what my natural hair really looks like due to a lifetime worth of dyes, relaxers, curling irons, and just plain abuse (and I didn't even know I was doing it) – like many of my fellow sisters, is sad. I was shocked to see how curly and soft, long and manageable my natural hair was. Had I stayed on the path that was all around me, I would've never known. We think we have to relax our hair because it is coarse, dry, and unruly; but this is because we've spent a countless amount of years altering it from its intended state – and it is, quite simply, weak and damaged. It is thirsty for moisture, and it's longing for proper nutrition, softer hands, less harsh chemicals, and overall proper care. Within only one year of giving my hair what it needs, it went from a short afro to longer than it's ever been in my life. There were no tricks needed, no chemicals, and no special pills – only a change of thinking. An alteration of perception in what I thought my hair was and its potential; and once my mind was there, the physical aspect followed. It was as simple as that. There are some who actually made the decision to go natural and have been for many years, yet are still not aware of what their hair needs to be healthy and blossom. These women have been left thinking that dry, coarse hair is all they could hope for. This is so very far from the truth. One example is a sister I found on a popular video-sharing website; she had been natural for over a decade with a dry, coarse, short afro that would never grow long or do anything but break. After reading up on the subject and gaining knowledge, her hair reached her bra strap within a year and a half. She had curls she'd never even seen in her hair before, and her hair was soft and manageable. Some people at this point, think, "Well that's her hair, not *my* hair." Well get ready, because it's your hair too. It doesn't matter how thick or coarse your hair presently is; it can thrive, grow, and be beautiful.

Many women who are natural have very strong opinions on the subject of women who have a relaxer, so let me start with this: This is not a militant book. It's not a book meant to bash any other race, creed or belief, nor is it meant to insult people who aren't natural. This book is only meant to let you know that you DO have a choice with your hair, and after you learn everything you need to on the subject, you may find that being natural is a choice you may actually want to go with. Many people relax their hair because to them, it's the only choice they have to look good and feel put together. And nothing is wrong with wanting to look your best; every woman should. Furthermore, every-one does things to "enhance their looks," if you will – from waxing your eyebrows to shaving to wearing makeup. I'm not knocking hair weaves, or anything else you may want to do to your hair. I wear braid extensions when I want to give my hair a break, and for protective styles. But are you doing it for a break or a change, or are you doing it because you believe your hair can't look good any other way? To know that black women are a minority, making up less than 10% of the population; yet despite these figures, according to industry statistics, we make up 34% of the $9 billion dollar hair care industry and over 60% of the hair weave industry (more, depending on which study you use), I think it's safe to say that black women spend a great deal of time and money altering the crown of their beauty from its original state, and we have to wonder why. Although many of us chalk it up to simple choice, the truth is, many of us believe that wearing our natural hair is not a feasible option, and we would not look as attractive in our own eyes if we did. The only thing I'm offering with this book is this: unlike what many may think, altering your natural state is not your only option for looking good or feeling beautiful. With this book, I want to give you the tools needed to transition your hair, nurture your hair, and allow it to reach its maximum potential.

Congratulations on taking the first step. Knowledge is power, so no matter where you go from here, it will be with the knowledge that God intended for you to have.

Mind Over Matter: The Significance of Hair and The Good Hair / Bad Hair Complex

So what is the big deal with hair, anyway? Why should it even matter what we do with our hair? It's just hair, right? Well, in my opinion, the answer is yes and no. In a simple breakdown, our hair is the crown of our head. The significance of hair dates way back to the Bible, the Qur'an, the Torah, and even Rastafarians. It signifies many things to many different people, but among them all, it mainly represents beauty, sensuality, strength, and even respect and energy. It is a part of our very being. The way we wear our hair definitely conveys a statement about our personality. Even making the choice to cut all of our hair off is a statement in itself. The health of our hair is also directly related to our frame of mind, stress levels, happiness, etc.

So what is the big deal? In my opinion, it's not what you do with your hair; it's more the reason behind the action(s). Many of us, from a very young age, have been led to believe that our hair isn't beautiful. We've been taught from an early age that it's ugly, it's 'nappy' (not even a negative term, but one that has been coined as such; 'nappy' simply means tightly-coiled hair), it looks and feels like Brillo®, and it doesn't grow. Some parents relax their children's hair as young as 6 years old and even younger. I am most grateful that my mother was not one of those people, but as a child, I felt very differently. Even though my mother didn't promote that type of thinking, it was all around me. My mother used to put my hair in braids, while all the other girls in school had perms, presses, jerry curls, etc. They (and I, in turn,) thought my hair was frizzy, big, and wouldn't lie down; and as far back as I can remember, I wanted my hair to look straight and "pretty," like everyone else. It was part of being accepted, and what child doesn't want that? The significance behind the thought that we have to change a part of ourselves just to feel accepted is sad. In fact, instead of looking at relaxers and weaves as a choice, many of us accept it as something we have to do to look pretty. What society deems as pretty and acceptable is a girl that has long, oftentimes straight hair; with a European, Latin or Indian type of texture. The closest we could get to that, in many women's eyes, was a relaxer. Then as time went on, we turned to wigs and extensions. Then weaves. And the closer they got to making the added hair look more like it's our own (lace wigs, bonding to your hair, glues, micros, etc.), the more expensive it became. And sadly, many women are happy to pay for it, to conform to what society deems as beautiful.

Do I wear extensions? Yes I do. I have nothing against them. For the first year of my big chop, the majority of the time, I wore braid extensions as a protective style because I didn't know how to care for my newfound strands yet, but I felt like if I braided it and left it alone, at least I couldn't do any damage to it and it would continue to grow in the meantime. I recently went away on vacation, and I knew I would be swimming and just doing a lot of things that my hair is not accustomed to on a daily basis; so I decided to put my hair in braids to protect it. I'm not big on weaves, but if you're wearing it to give your hair a break or as a protective style or even a just a change, that's more than fine. The problem comes in when you think that's all you can do with your hair, because wearing your own hair feels, to you, like it's not "done," or it's unkempt, or it's just plain ugly – and why would you wear your own 'ugly' hair when you could just buy yourself some 'new' hair, right? But here's the thing: Who decided that our hair was ugly? Who set the standard that relaxing our hair was so much better than our beautiful, natural hair? Who decided that Caucasian hair, Spanish hair, Indian hair, or any other culture's hair for that matter, was better than ours? We are a beautiful, colorful race with an endless variety of beauty that doesn't need to be altered. If we only took the time to discover our own beauty, instead of focusing on changing the very core of who we are, I think that we would be much better off. Some people may tell you that it depends on your hair type if you should go natural, and imply that if your hair has a tighter curl, it cannot be beautiful if worn natural. How ridiculous. What kind of hair you were born with is part of what makes you, ***you***. How can that not be beautiful? Some of us have fine, wavy hair. Some of us have big, thick curly tendrils. Some of us have really tight, coily curls that are springy and bouncy. Some of us have hair that is puffy, soft, and plentiful. ALL of us have beautiful hair that is versatile and able to grow long, strong, and healthy – if we'd only learn how to care for it.

But where did the good hair/bad hair state of mind begin? Many would say that it started in slavery days. Our hair was in need of care at that time because we were not provided, of course, with the tools needed to groom ourselves – picks and larger combs weren't needed for the Caucasian people that brought us here, and were considered weapons. The masters leaned towards choosing "house" slaves whose hair looked more like their masters; or if not, they were instructed to either keep their hair very low, covered, or straightened with a straightening comb. The "good hair" concept was not about our hair being bad, but actually an opportunity to live a little better life in the house, instead of working in the fields. After slavery, this concept still continued, with women with straighter hair being chosen for work and deemed more acceptable looking than those with natural hair. The ones that had a straighter or mixed texture were deemed ones that had "good hair," with natural-haired black women having bad hair. This actually continued for a very long time, to some degree. In 1971, a news reporter, Melba Tolliver, made national news when she covered the wedding of the daughter of President Nixon while wearing an afro. The news station was not pleased and threatened to fire her, until the story became national news. As recent as 1981, another news reporter, Dorothy Reed, was suspended for wearing her hair in braids with beads on the air. The news station called her hairstyle "inappropriate and distracting." After public scrutiny and the NAACP intervening, however, the station allowed her to return back to work with back pay, and she came back with her braids, just minus the beads. When you hear about these types of battles that black women took on just to be themselves and not conform to what another culture has deemed acceptable for them, it's surprising that we still regard our own hair so negatively.

So based on history, we know that their version of "good hair" was completely wrong, and just meant to have us look more like them.

What is it really, then? I personally don't like the term at all. But if someone asked me to define it, I would say "good hair" is groomed hair. Clean hair. Hair that is done and neat. It has nothing to do with the texture, wave, curl, or lack thereof. It has to do with you being presentable, and taking care of yourself.

Many relaxed women take a huge offense to naturals making statements that women who wear perms or weaves display self-hatred. This is a very touchy subject, and I think making such a general statement is very extreme. But I think this all goes back, once again, to your intentions. I don't think that women who have a perm sit around hating themselves; to many, a perm is just the normal thing to do without a lot of thought put into it at all, except the desire to have straight and smooth hair. It doesn't automatically mean low self-esteem if women have a perm, or that women automatically love themselves more if they don't have a perm, for that matter. Weaves can just be a protective style, a color option, or just simply a change. With that said, however, whether we realize it or not, when we believe that altering our hair is not just an option, but based on a belief that we don't have a choice because what we were born with isn't a good option, there is an unconscious statement that we are making – and we are passing this thinking on to our children.

If you think I'm wrong, consider this: If you saw a Caucasian, Indian, or Latin woman wearing a weave that was an Afro-textured, kinky Afro, what would you think? I mean, she likes herself, it's just her choice because she likes her hair to look like black women's hair, and she has the right to look any way she wants, right? But many of you would not think of it that way at all. Yet it's perfectly acceptable for us to walk around with weaves of other races' hair textures. What do you think the reason is for that? Is our hair not the hair to be desired for someone to weave into their hair? I wonder why? Could it be because the general thinking is our hair is not as 'nice' as others? This is not to disparage or spread hate about another race, just to spread love for our own. Why do we relax our hair, really? Some will say, "It's not that I don't like my hair, it's just my CHOICE, and I have that right." And for some, that may very well be true and is perfectly fine. We are ALL entitled to choice, and should live our lives as we see fit. But for others, I can say that I have known people throughout my life that feel as if wearing their own natural hair is absolutely absurd.

"It's way too nappy"

"I wouldn't be able to do anything with it"

"Maybe YOU have hair that you can go natural and work with, but I DON'T."

This is not made up words. It's words that I've heard over and over again. A mental thinking that wearing your own hair is not even an option, and this is really sad. When I see children feeling bad because their hair isn't straightened like the other kids and feeling ugly inside, that is very disheartening. Or even worse, a child not seeing anything wrong with their hair, but parents telling them that it looks bad and needs to be relaxed. Children being taken to the beautician as early as 6 years old or younger to get a relaxer, how could that not be all they ever know? How could they not think that obviously their hair is not "good" enough, if we're altering it at such a young age?

A guy I know once told me that he lived with his child's mother for 5 or 6 years, and he had never seen her real hair. NEVER. How is that even possible? You live with someone and you've never seen her hair? But she wouldn't let him. She said it was too 'nappy,' and she refused to let him see her that way, even when he tried. According to him, she simply wanted to always look her best. So in her eyes, her "best" had to be with a weave? I believe in my heart that something is seriously wrong with that kind of thinking.

So what do we do? Do we have a responsibility to teach our children differently? I think we do. Does that mean you have to go natural? It would be nice, but no. Just making it clear to the children in your life that relaxing their hair is a choice, not a necessity – I think is a very good route to take. Letting them know that they are beautiful – natural or relaxed – and learning how to care for their hair so it isn't so unmanageable is a great option. Some people say the craziest things in front of their children and don't even realize the impact it's making:

"I don't know why you couldn't have hair like your sister's"

"This hair is so nappy!"

"We need to get you a perm quick!"

"Now SHE has good hair."

Letting our children know that they are beautiful *just the way they are* is a crucial step in building up our children's self-esteem and pride in themselves. Let's all make a conscious effort to do this.

Mind Over Matter: Acceptance

The Workplace: Many bring up the subject of wearing a relaxer for their profession. And this is a very real and valid concern. After all, how many naturals are in your office? Wow. Just saying that out loud is sad. We feel like we have to alter our appearance to be more successful – not because we're not happy with what we were born with, but because we have accepted that in order to get ahead in certain careers, we have to look more like another race, and less like ourselves. People believe that the corporate world will not embrace them if they wear their natural hair. And at one time (not too long ago, in fact), this was very true.

Well, thankfully, we don't live in that time anymore. Speaking from my own experience and the experiences of women I've encountered: Although there are those ignorant few that still exist and will try to bring you down (I have not encountered any, but I am not ignorant to their existence), I can honestly say that I have received more acceptance and compliments from fellow colleagues (men and women) in my office, Caucasians, other races, and people from other countries than even my own race. That is a fact. In the society we live in today, natural hair is much more accepted than the days of the past, and unlike what many people picture in their minds when they think of natural hair, natural hair is not limited to an afro (though there's absolutely nothing wrong with that either). Your natural hair can be very neat, stylish, and well put together for the workplace. It's difficult for me to even fathom how natural hair could be regarded as a less-professional look than weaves that don't fit a woman's natural features, or that are way, way over the top in terms of style, quantity and colors. But this book is not about bashing (smile).

Back to my previous point – sad to say, I have had my own people down me more than any other race when I first started going natural. Some would ask, "So you're just doing this for a while so your hair could stop breaking, then you're going to perm it, right?" Or, "Oh, you're going natural? When you perm it again, it's going to look so nice!" I once had a black man, a friend of mine, straight ask me, "But what are you going to do about the 'nappies'?" Ha! He had a straight face and everything. Oftentimes in today's society, you have to worry MORE about acceptance from your friends and family than a job or a profession. Sad, but true. There are natural-haired bankers, models, people in the corporate world, actresses, singers, athletes, accountants, and more. As a matter of fact, if you look on TV these days, you might be hard pressed to find a commercial with a black woman that has a weave or relaxer, because the majority of them are using women with natural hair of all hair types (not just a finer or mixed texture). The professional world is not going to be your worst enemy, and for the most part, going natural is not going to be a deal-breaker either.

Your Friends and Family: This particular area is a really tough one, because no one wants to be ridiculed by the people they love. It's disheartening and hurtful. You would think something like how you wear your hair would not be that big a deal. Not so. Many may not approve of your decision to go natural, and some may not be shy about letting you know their opinions, either. Some will question why you are doing this. Others will look with disapproving eyes, and some with worrying eyes. Let's start with the fact that when it comes to family, like parents for instance, they generally just want what they think is best for you. Some are concerned about how people may react to your decision, how you will be accepted in the corporate world, etc. Some have been brought up in a time when this was not at all acceptable and our people did everything to "blend in" and not be alienated, so it is possible that they are just genuinely concerned for you. Although this is no longer the case, this reaction is sometimes due to a lack of knowledge about natural hair, and sometimes, an out-of-touch perspective on recent times; combined with the in-bred, negative thinking regarding what our hair represents. Back when your parents were growing up (depending on their age), natural hair in the corporate world was in fact a big deal, and that might be basically all they know. Because of this, please try to exercise patience when defending your decision. Try educating them and reassuring them, as opposed to being defensive. This solution can be more productive for the both of you.

Friends usually other befriend people that have their same interests and similar personalities. When you go outside of the normal realm of this, people tend to shy away from the unknown. In either case, don't be angry with them, and try not to get defensive. Just calmly let them know your reasoning behind your decision, inform them of the dangers of the harsh chemicals from relaxers or your need to embrace your natural self, or whatever your own personal reasons are for going natural. Please try to be patient with them and know that your decision is just that – *yours*. There's no need to fight a battle you've already won; it's your hair, it doesn't really matter WHAT they say, so be pleasant when telling them how you feel. Above everything else, know that your parents or anyone else in your family, or your circle of friends, are not you. You have to make decisions for yourself, and if they're really your friends and family, they will come around eventually. Or, at the very least, you can agree to disagree.

Your Partner: Admittedly, partners are very different from your family or friends. I knew a girl who was natural, and she told me she had to end up relaxing her hair because her husband hated it. He told her she needed to do something with her hair because he was "tired of her walking around looking like that." I will not speak on or judge her husband, but I imagine that had to hurt. I will say that she readily admitted that she just didn't know how to care for it, so it was oftentimes dry, felt coarse, and never really looked neat, so in the end, she just gave up. What a bad place to find yourself in. You've made the choice to go natural and embrace your natural beauty, but now, you're lost as to what to do next. You're frustrated and ready to give up, and your partner's confused and not sure where this is going; what do you do? This is the very reason for this book. To make sure that every woman who picks this book up will not be in this unfortunate situation.

Because your hair is a definite representation of you, no matter how you look at it, even though the final decision is still yours, going natural is definitely something you should discuss with your significant other. I had that talk with my boyfriend during that time, especially since the beginning is definitely the hardest part of the transition. There were days when he would walk into my room and although he didn't say anything, he'd have his eyebrows up, like, "Where is this going??" I would smile and tell him, "Just be patient, honey; it won't be like this for long." He would reply, unsurely, "OK!" But he did remain patient. And he quickly saw that his patience was not in vain. I'm not saying that this isn't a major transition, but chances are, if he loves you, he'll love you just the same. You can choose to transition with wigs, braids, or other hairstyles like twist outs, or you could be brave and cut it all off. Either way you go, know that although we're all individuals, in all fairness, it will be a huge change for your significant other, and one that he deserves a little time to prepare himself for, so try to keep that in mind.

Finally, there are other people that are not against natural hair, but when they think of people who are natural, they think of afros, picks, puffs, and the like; and although nothing is wrong with this at all, it's simply just not their style. Well the truth is, the possibilities with natural hair don't end there, they are endless. You can wear so many hairstyles, it's truly amazing. It actually opens up a whole new world of styles for us that we could not do when our hair was bone straight. You can keep your hair natural and still have a neat appearance. You can keep your hair natural and still be fashion-forward. You can wear your natural hair and look absolutely beautiful. You just have to change your thinking, and open your mind to the possibilities.

Mind over Matter: How Do Black Men Really Feel About Women With Natural Hair?

This topic comes up so often that I had to discuss it briefly. In my personal opinion, because of the media and society, many of our black men need to relearn the definition of beauty and know that we don't have to alter ourselves to be beautiful. But to be fair to them, I think there are misconceptions out there with Black women on how a great deal Black men really feel about women with natural hair, and it has been the deciding factor for many, many women to opt against going natural. No one wants to be unattractive to the opposite sex, and there's nothing wrong with that. But maybe we need to look a little further.

I've watched countless videos online, performed research in social media outlets, read articles, and asked my own male friends and colleagues how they felt about this topic. These men are from all walks of life, different locations, ages, and backgrounds, and this is what the majority of black men had to say about the subject:

The word most spoken from almost all of them (literally almost all) is "confidence." This word was spoken in many different contexts, and I will break them all down here:

• Most of the men felt that a woman that is natural exudes a certain confidence about herself. They feel like it tells them a lot about her character and what kind of woman she is. This is very attractive to many of the men.

• That same confidence, however, is the reason some men gave for many black men not approaching a woman with natural hair (weird). Time and time again, I heard them say that some men won't talk to a natural-haired woman because they feel like she knows she has it going on. She is confident and she is strong, and that in itself may be intimidating for some men. Similar to a woman with very short hair, they feel in order to pull that off, a woman has to be very confident in who she is, and some men may not be brave enough to approach her. They insisted that it was not because they didn't like the concept of natural hair.

• Some men don't understand what the big deal is either way; for them, hair is hair. In their eyes, they're looking for more than hair, and as long as you're confident (there's that word again) in whatever hair you have, natural hair would not make them less attracted to you.

• Many men talked about how you wear the hair (not referring to style, rather, your confidence). When you are self-conscious about your hair or don't personally think it looks good, it shows, and it isn't attractive. But if you are confident about your hair, even when it's really short, that's what makes it so attractive. So if you're going to wear your hair natural, do it with confidence. Experiment until you find styles that *you* think looks good on you, so that you can wear them well. The spark that a woman gives off when she walks down the street with her hair, her clothes, her shoes, everything; when she's confident, it shows, and men are very attracted to that.

• Almost everyone dispelled the idea that they think of a natural woman as too afro-centric, or militant, or anything of the kind (not that anything is wrong with being afro-centric). They said it would have to be more than her hair that gives off that impression (for instance, her clothes). They would not think she was too afro-centric, for example, if she had natural hair with high heels and a really nice dress on, earrings, etc. When they think of militant or afro-centric, they think of an afro, with no makeup at all or void of any grooming; plain clothes, and not very feminine. They also mentioned things like shells in the hair and beads as "going over the top" (their words, ladies, not mine).

• This point was the most negative thing I heard about natural hair. Many of the men felt their dislike had nothing to do with natural hair, but it had more to do with hair that was not being taken cared of. They like natural hair, but they don't like to see dry (many used the word "dry") hair that looks uncombed and unkempt, like the woman didn't do anything to it at all before leaving the house. Besides needing you to look like you're well put together next to them, they like the idea of being able to put their hands in a woman's hair. If your hair looks dry and not taken cared of, it's not attractive to them. These same men have insisted it has nothing to do with what type of hair you have, because they've seen women with kinky or short hair that take care of their hair, or hair that has dreads, twists, braids or Bantu knots, and if it was taken cared of, they liked it. They had no problem with curly hair, thick hair, or puffy hair; it just has to look like it's being taken cared of: clean, neat, combed, and soft; not looking as if it was just left to knot up (like a nappy fro) and feel dry (a few mentioned that the some women's hair looked like it needed more conditioning). They also mentioned they didn't like too much gel, grease, or hair adornments (beads, etc.) In short, they basically liked hair that was "welcoming" to be touched. I had one man tell me with no apologies that he did not think that natural hair was for "everyone," because of the same reasons above (he, incidentally, was dating a natural-haired woman at the time, but she had approximately 3A-B hair). He felt like some women, because of the texture of their hair, could not hope for anything more than that type of dry, unkempt-looking hair, and they should not go natural because they could never get that clean, neat, put-together look. When I shared with him my thoughts about women learning how to care for their new natural hair and shared some examples to him, he was much more open to the idea of every woman being able to go natural. But I appreciated his honesty, and am sure that he is not the only man that feels this way.

• A few of the men mentioned that they have an attraction to long hair. They didn't care if it was natural or permed, just long (long being shoulder-length or longer). They did not like the idea of being with a woman whose hair was as short as theirs. They did add that if it was her BC (Big Chop) and she had to do it to go natural, they would deal with that stage – just as long as it didn't stay that way.

• Almost every single black man, in every different form of re-search I conducted, said they do not like weaves. They could deal with braids, twists, or anything else, but disliked weaves. It is very unattractive to them, and they don't like the feel or even look of them. Not to mention the feeling that it gives them – that the woman is fake, or is not confident enough with her own hair or looks (many also mentioned too much makeup in the same sentence). These are their words – different men in different conversations and mediums. When asked, "Why then, do men always date women with weaves?" They contended that they don't have a choice and have accepted it as the norm; so many women now wear weaves that it would seriously cut their female selection pool down to nil if they made that stand. But it is not their choice. It is, as a matter of fact, their last choice. WOW. That was very interesting to me. My own ex-husband despised weaves, wigs or anything of the kind. I think that our perception, based on the media and the world we live in, has misguided us into thinking that a great deal of things we spend money on matter to men; when in fact, it doesn't, or they may not even like it.

Now that I have written what came from them, I will write my own thoughts on the subject:

I admit that I am not a man, and I can't speak for them. But I can speak about my own experiences, which are similar to other women's experiences that I've known. And I can say that it is our experiences *why* we feel that men think a certain way. I'm not saying that what they're saying about being attracted to natural-haired girls is not true. It just doesn't seem to show very much. Which is the part that's most confusing, because I can honestly say that my natural hair is literally a "man magnet" for Caucasian men, as well as other races. Strange, crazy, I know – but absolutely true. Men of other races who would have never looked at me before (especially Caucasian men) are so very drawn to me now that my hair is natural. It actually took me a while to figure out what it was, then it hit me and was confirmed. Some will actually reach out while talking to me and touch my hair. It's unbelievable. When I'm around my own black men, however, when my natural hair was growing out, I never got that same intensity. Not that men weren't attracted to me, but it almost felt to me that it was despite the hair, not because of it (or not because the hair played a positive part). Sometimes I just got crazy with my natural hair and wore it wild and free, or experimented with Mohawks and such when I was going out, then paired the look with high heels and dressy clothes, which gave off a certain aura that they were attracted to (I guess confirming the "confident" statements), but when I just wore my natural hair in braids, twists, or even in a bun on a normal day, it was not the same attention as my relaxed hair at all. It was only after my hair grew long that black men started complimenting my hair often, and seemed to be very drawn to it. I definitely agree that they love long hair, but when it was short or the average length and natural, not so much. So to hear them say it's attractive to them is kind of hard for me to swallow. I did have one experience that made me think a little differently. I met a handsome, very nice man a while back who, when asked what he thought of me when he first met me, said the first thing he noticed was my natural hair, and it was very attractive to him. I honestly would have never known that if I wasn't told, because he never said anything to me, and my general thinking was as I just mentioned. Which goes to show that I obviously don't know what goes on in their heads, and maybe I should just ask. I also never thought about being intimidated as a reason for not approaching a natural-haired woman. So what are we to do about that? I really don't know. But I do know that knowledge is power, so maybe just the thought of knowing that going natural is not a negative to many of them is helpful. Take from it what you will, ladies.

Understanding: Hair Structure, Textures, Types and Conditions

If you're now ready to go natural and make such a big change to your hair, you'll first need to understand what is needed for the hair to thrive and be at its best in a natural state. Let's start by understanding our hair structure and why it seems that black hair can't "grow" (I use that word loosely, but we'll get into that later).

First, the basic breakdown of a strand. We'll start from the inside and work our way out, only breaking down the parts vital to individual hair care:

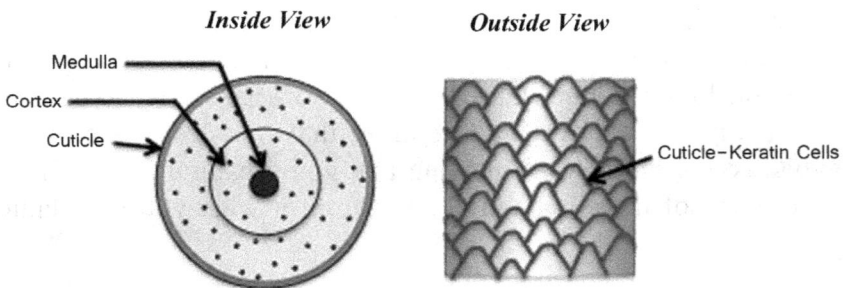

Inside View   *Outside View*

Medulla
Cortex
Cuticle
Cuticle–Keratin Cells

The cortex is near the center of the hair, and inside is the Medulla (the very core of your hair shaft). The cortex contains the natural pigment of your hair (melanin), and is what provides the hair with strength, elasticity, and its texture. This is why it's most important to feed your hair the proper nutrients, not just coat the outside to make it look shiny temporarily; or what you may actually be doing is weighing the hair down and blocking the hair from absorbing the proper nutrients.

The cuticle is the outer layer of the hair shaft. It is made up of overlapping transparent keratin cells, or what is commonly referred to as scales, that serve as a protective barrier. A healthy cuticle state is when the cells are laying down and the hair feels smooth, but not tight enough where nutrients cannot be absorbed. The cuticle's job is to protect the cortex from outside forces, like heat and chemical breakdowns. This is also the part of your hair that determines its smoothness, softness and shine, because a) it gets coated with sebum, and b) if the cells (or scales) are healthy and lying down, it will reflect more light, and will feel smooth to the touch. The cuticle can get damaged from harsh chemicals like perms and relaxers, too much heat, brushing and combing your hair too much or too vigorously, and too much chlorine in swimming pools.

In the scalp:

The hair follicle is the part of the skin that 'grows' the hair. The average rate of hair growth on a scalp with healthy hair follicles is approximately a half an inch per month.

And finally, the sebaceous glands (attached to the hair follicle) produce the sebum that coats the hair and conditions it naturally. Have you ever had a wash and set or even a perm, and felt like you needed a day or two for the hair to look its best? That's because by then, the sebum has traveled down the hair shaft again and reconditioned it, making it look shiny and healthy. Sebum is an oily substance mostly made up of good fats, wax, keratin, and cellular material. The thicker your hair is, the more sebaceous glands you have.

Hair Textures

So, what is the difference between Caucasian hair (or even Indian, Spanish, and other cultures) and black hair? First things first: Black people have the most variety of hair than any other race. Therefore, it is virtually impossible to put us in specific categories, because the amount of categories we would have would be endless. But in general, broad terms, there are some very basic differences that distinguish people of an African origin from our counterparts.

Asian Hair   Caucasian Hair   Black Hair

Hair is generally broken down into three groups:

Asian hair, Caucasian hair, and Black hair.

Straight hair has a round hair follicle, while wavy hair has an oval follicle.

The curlier the hair, the flatter the hair follicle. The flatter the hair follicle, the weaker the hair.

Believe it or not, ASIAN hair is, on average, the thickest of all three kinds of hair. It also grows the fastest, is the least dense (the amount of hairs on the head), and has the most elasticity. Asian hair is almost always straight, with circular follicles throughout their cross-sections (we'll get more into cross-sections later). Their hair is so thick, it's not very easy to alter. This is not always good for styling and can be frustrating, but like all hair, it has a beauty of its own.

Caucasian hair can have a few hair types: it can be straight, wavy, or even curly hair. The hair follicle is round and can be circular or slightly oval-shaped in the cross sections. Also, each hair is almost always thinner than Asian or Black hair. A Black hair strand can be up to three times thicker than a Caucasian's.

Now we can talk about cross-sections (also called cross-bonds) so you can understand:

Black Hair is generally almost always coiled or spiraled. Generally speaking, a black hair follicle is oval in shape (not round). Our hair is the only hair that is shaped like this. Also, the cross sections in black hair, instead of staying a consistent shape, gets flatter in the cross sections; depending on your hair type, it can get flatter to the point of being almost completely flat and thin (like a string of ribbon). This cross section is where the hair kinks (or bends if you will), and the constant alternating between the rounder oval and the flatter oval sections is how the hair forms your coil, or your spiraled curl. This also means that your hair is considerably stronger in the thicker, rounder hair sections, and weaker in the flatter cross sections, where the hair forms the bend for your curl. This is why the thinner your hair is at the cross sections or even the more cross-sections you may have, the tighter your curl, AND the more delicate your hair is and drier your hair can be; which in turn makes it prone to breakage if you don't know how to care for it. This is why black people with naturally straighter hair or with a gene "mix" if you will (that causes the textures in their hair to be straighter than most ethnic women), appears to be able to grow longer hair easier with less breakage than people with curlier hair or tightly-coiled hair. Notice I said "easier" – not that having curly hair makes it impossible to attain growth by any stretch.

Now that we understand the differences in our hair from other races, we are now ready for our first step: to begin to understand and accept the fact that we cannot care for our hair the same way that other races do, or continually alter our hair to be like other races without repercussions. Because our hair is has a totally different makeup, we have to simply change our thought process on what we knew was right to care for our hair, as our hair has its own special needs and should be cared for totally differently. Altering your natural hair temporarily (heat styles, etc.) is acceptable, as long as it's not done often; but a permanent alteration of your hair chemically, for any race, can definitely have repercussions.

Hair Types

Let's talk about the different hair types for black hair. Like I said before, Black people have the most varying hair types than any other race. Our beautiful race spans from one end of the gene pool to the other. This is why it's very hard to group our hair into 4 categories. Even in one person's individual head of hair, it is very common for a black person to have two types of hair, or even three types.

There's a word I will be mentioning in this section and throughout the book that I just want to touch on: "shrinkage." It's a word you've never really used to describe hair, but when you become natural, the word becomes a term that will be very common in your conversations. When we think of the word shrinkage, we think of something actually shrinking. But, to everyone's relief, natural hair doesn't actually shrink. It just that because our hair is so curly, it appears shorter than it actually is. Therefore, the tighter (smaller) our curls are, the more "shrinkage" we will have. The looser your curl, the more the hair hangs down and displays more length, but the tighter your curl, the more the hair springs upward, making the hair appear much shorter than it really is. Depending on your hair type, some people can have up to 70% shrinkage. WOW. That's a lot. I don't personally know anyone that has that much shrinkage, but the reality is, having any type of curly hair means that you will have to deal with some percentage of shrinkage (personally, my hair is a little past my collarbone when curly, and past the middle of my back – below my bra strap – when straight) which can definitely take some getting used to. This is sometimes why some people lean towards straightening their natural hair – they want to be able to show off their actual length. There's nothing wrong with doing this every once in a while, just be careful to exercise the proper care when doing so, and know that the more you do it, the more prone you are to heat damage, or your hair not reverting back to its curls in random places because of that damage.

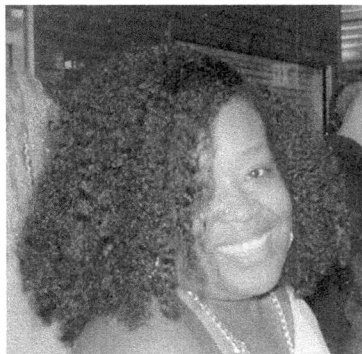

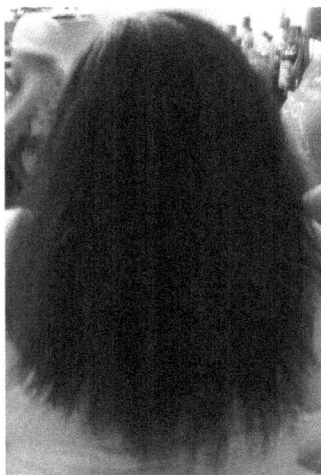

Shrinkage: This curly hair that's a little past my shoulders is really this length when straight, past the middle of my back.

Hair texture is basically your hair's thickness, and at the risk of being too general, we will say that it will generally be in one of three categories: Fine, Medium, or Thick.

The Density of your hair is not about how thick the strands are, but how many hairs you actually have on your head. Once again, for the sake of putting it in categories, we'll say they generally fall in three – Sparse (less than the average amount of hair on your head), Medium (about average), and High (more than the average amount of hair on your head).

Now we will get into the hair types. Our genes determine what our hair type will be. The average black women's hair typically falls in the Type 2-4 Categories, with more concentration in 3 and 4; but because we have so much variety in our race, I will break them all down. If you're trying to determine your hair type from this guide, the best way to see your curl pattern is to first wash and condition your hair, preferably with natural or very gentle products. Reason being: a) you can see your curls better when your hair is wet, and

b) the natural products help your hair's PH to be balanced, and that allows your curls to pop. Many people are under the misconception that your hair type has to do with how thick or coarse your hair is. This is very untrue. You have people who have fine hair or thick, dense hair have the same hair type. The hair type has to do with your curl, wave, or lack thereof:

Hair Types

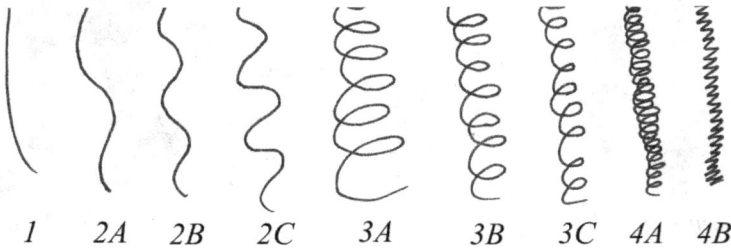

1   2A   2B   2C   3A   3B   3C   4A   4B

Type 1 Hair: Type 1 hair is completely straight. There is no curl pattern to it at all, no change in the cross sections (or cross-bonds) as previously mentioned. Most black women do not have this hair type, but with our beautiful wide variety of features, it is worth mentioning. Type 1 hair, unless damaged, tends to look shinier (and therefore appears healthier) than wavy or curly hair. This is not because it is so, rather it is because there are no curls or bends in the hair, so light is able to reflect better on it. If Type 1 hair is not shiny and has a dull appearance, it can either be dirty, or damaged.

Type 2 Hair: All the hair in the Type 2 section refer to loose, wavy hair. Women of many races fall under this category, including black women. It has a natural "S" pattern, and hangs to show more of its length. It is also easily straightened. There are three types in this category, but all with the same attributes as described here.

2A hair is very fine, wavy hair and thin in texture. The waves are very, very loose in this type. It is very easy to handle; and is very easily straightened or curled.

2B hair is medium-textured, wavy hair and little more resistant to different styles. The waves are a little deeper, and it can also have a tendency to be frizzy.

2C hair is thicker in texture, even more resistant to styling, and has an even greater tendency to frizz. The waves are very deep, and much more defined.

Type 3 Hair is where you'll begin to find more black women (although we are definitely in Type 2 as well). This type of hair coils and looks more like ringlets, as opposed to type 2's wavy pattern (think Shirley Temple curls). Type 3 hair usually has a lot of body and the hair is very bouncy and springy. It has more shrinkage than Type 2, but less than type 4, and has the ability to hang with the right manipulation. It is usually very soft if taken cared of, and although it is a lot of hair, it can also be very fine in texture, just dense. Most people with this type of hair find it easier to wear their natural hair in its normal state. They also oftentimes have a combination of Type 3 curls in one head of hair, or even a bit of Type 4 as well. The three hair types break down like this:

3A hair tends to have large ringlets that naturally hang when loose, and the hair looks shinier than other type 3s. The size of the curls itself can be like the width of a fat piece of colored chalk.

3B hair has medium-size ringlets, and is also very bouncy. They don't hang as much as 3A, but the curls are very defined and may be the size of your index finger, with the curl pattern noticeable from a reasonable distance.

3C hair has tighter curls, much like a corkscrew, or the width of a pencil. The hair texture in this type can go from very fine to very thick. Most people with this hair type have dense hair, with a great deal of curls on one head that make it time-consuming to alter or style.

Type 4 Hair is much kinkier than the other types. Many people have the misconception that 'kinky' hair means hair that is hard to the touch or hard to comb. Kinky simply means hair that it is tightly coiled or curled. Although Type 4 hair is very tightly coiled, it can still have a very defined pattern that is clearly displayed. Most people think this hair is the thickest. On the contrary: because of the many crosshairs that make up the tight coils, Type 4 hair is actually often finer than the other types in texture, and needs special attention, due to its fragility. It can also, however, be very thick, with an abundance of hair on one head packed in together. This type of hair also has the least amount of cuticle layers, which adds to its vulnerable state if cared for with rough hands (forceful combing and brushing), excessive heat, or chemicals. Because of the tightest coils of any other hair type, this type of hair shrinks the most – shrinking up to 70% of its actual hair length (depending on what you read, some say even more). I know of a girl who has type 4B hair: when in its natural state, her hair is at her shoulders. When she straightens it, however, it is on her stomach near her belly button. This hair has two only types:

4A hair is very tightly coiled, but still has a curly, defined ringlet pattern like type 3s. 4A's curls can be as tight as the width of a hairpin. Generally, they are a little bigger than that.

4B hair no longer has a ringlet pattern. When stretched, 4B hair actually looks more like a "Z" than an "S." From far away, it is difficult to see any pattern at all. This type of hair, when cared for, is actually quite soft, and feels similar to a big ball of cotton. This hair tends to hold in less moisture than the previous types, and needs to be cared for with gentle hands, lots of conditioner, and little chemicals.

As I mentioned earlier, it is very common for a woman to have two or even three different types of hair on their head. I have three types of hair on my head, with a section of my hair that is more prone to dryness than the rest (it's in the middle, on the top of my head). Because I am aware of it, I take special care to moisturize it a little bit more than the rest, I pay more attention to the ends of the hair in that section, and I put a little bit more product in that section as well. Because of this special care, the average person would never even notice that it is different from the rest of my hair, but I know, and I have learned to give it what it needs to look and feel its best.

Hair Condition

Coarse/Wiry Hair

People tend to confuse thick hair for coarse hair, because thick hair is prone to coarseness more than the other hair textures. However, coarse hair is NOT a hair type, but a condition. (REPEAT it in your head). It can happen to thick, medium, or any type of dry hair. Coarse hair happens when the outside layers (or scales of your hair) are raised up at the shaft, instead of laying down smooth. This gives the hair a rough feeling to the touch; and because the hair layers are raised and therefore open, it can't seal or lock in the moisture – so no matter how much you moisturize it, it seems to always revert back to dry hair in no time (this is when your hair is in a porous condition). If your hair is prone to this condition, if you don't take the time to moisturize and deep condition the hair on a constant, regular basis, coarse, dry and brittle hair will be the result. However, with the correct care and handling, hair that you thought could never feel anything but coarse, can feel smooth and soft to the touch.

Understanding: The Relaxing Process

Some people wonder what the big deal really is in relaxing your hair in the first place. Let me start by saying everyone is entitled to choice, and it's your hair. I just think that it's important to know all of the facts of a situation before you make a sound decision:

Over 80% of the dry weight of your hair is made up of the protein keratin. Keratin contains a large amount of disulfide, from an amino acid called cysteine in your hair. It is your disulfide bonds (also called 'cross-sections' or 'cross-bonds') that make your hair curly. The more cross-sections you have, the curlier your hair will be. Now what relaxers do, in order to make your hair straight, is penetrate the outer layer of your hair and go into the cortex layer (the inner layer), and break down these cross-sections, then cap them so that they cannot reform. Sodium Hydroxide is the chemical that is found in lye relaxers. It is the strongest type of chemical used in relaxers because it breaks down the cross-sections the most effectively (it is also found in drain cleaner, by the way). The PH factor of relaxers with Sodium Hydroxide ranges from 10 to 13, based on the strength you buy and how much is in the relaxer. Our normal, healthy hair's PH should be within the range of 4.5 and 5.5. Now let me put this in perspective for you. The total range of PH is from a 0 (strongly Acidic) to 14 (Strongly Alkaline). So the relaxer is near the highest point on the scale. The internet indicates that Depilatories (hair removers) work by "breaking down the disulfide bonds in keratin and weakening the hair, so that it is easily scraped off where it emerges from the hair follicle." Hmmm. Sound familiar? Most hair removers are at a PH of 14. If a relaxer is only ONE PH point from literally breaking the hair down so it "easily scrapes off" of your head, don't you think you're playing with the health of your hair (and your scalp for that matter) every time you use a relaxer? No-lye relaxer (made with Guanidine Hydroxide), although not as strong, has the same exact job as the previous Hydroxide: to break down the cross-sections, damaging the inner part of your hair and capping them so they do not reform. It has to be strong enough to accomplish this, so it is still very strong.

This is why there is a need for a neutralizing shampoo after a re-laxer: to try to lower the PH. If not, the hair can actually swell and break off. If you've ever known anyone whose hair literally just broke off after a perm, it was because the hair's PH was so high, it could not withstand it, and it broke off of their head. Wow. This is serious stuff that we are doing to alter our hair. Is it worth it?

Many will argue that they know many women whose hair is very healthy and pretty with a perm, so I obviously don't know what I'm talking about. To them, I say to please ponder this: every normal woman's hair, no matter the ethnicity, continually grows. You can find proof of this in the fact that every month or two, you need a touch up for your relaxer if you have one, correct? What are we doing when we get a touch up? Relaxing the 'new growth,' right? So this would stand to reason that like every other race, black hair continually grows. Now knowing this, if your hair is continually growing and "healthy," why is it the average black women's hair only reaches shoulder length and no longer? Where does all that hair growth go? Many of us believe our hair only "grows" to our shoulders, but this is far from the truth, otherwise you would have no new growth to have to relax – your hair would simply grow to a certain length and stop. It would then stand to reason that if it's continually growing but not getting any longer, then many black women are not retaining their length. Why? Because of a fact most of us don't stop to ponder: it is actually breaking off. Before going natural, my hair was about shoulder length all my life. And as long as it looked shiny and the ends were cut, I thought it was healthy. I went natural and some months later, did my big chop in February. By November of the following year, exactly 1 year and 9 months later, my hair was at my bra strap down the middle of my back. Did it begin to grow at a superhuman speed that it never grew before? No. I was just able to actually retain the length that it was growing, because it was strong and healthy. Something that a perm never allowed me to do, because it weakened my hair. Can some people still grow long hair with a relaxer? Sure. But for the vast majority, we all know the answer to that question is no. Absolutely not, as a matter of fact. Anything past our collar bone, people begin to wonder "Where did she get all that hair from? Is she mixed?" It's a reality that we've lived with every day. All I'm offering is another way. A healthier way. A way where you can see and feel just how beautiful, long, and strong your own hair can be. Worse-case scenario? Your hair grows and gets back strong, and you can then relax it if you don't like it. You have nothing to actually lose.

Getting Down To Business: Cutting it All Off
(The Big Chop)

For some, choosing to cut off all of their relaxed hair instead of transitioning as the hair grows out (what is termed as the "Big Chop" or the "BC") can be the most freeing, liberating experience. But to be able to cut off all of your hair and still feel beautiful and secure about your looks, for others, can be a big feat.

Some say you have to be skinny. Some say you have to have the right shaped face or even head. Some say you have to have the right kind of texture of hair, so the hair can lie down as it's growing. The truth is, I've seen skinny girls, big girls, tall girls and short girls, girls with really tight, coily hair, and girls with fine, wavy hair – all cut their hair off and look amazing. I don't think it has to do with your size, shape, hair texture or anything else but the fact that if you're going to cut it, you're going to have to wear it with confidence.

There are some people who can put on something totally outside of the norm, but because of the way they wear it – with style, confidence, and flair – they make people fall in love with it, even if it may not be what they normally would have cared for. This is many times how new fashions are born.

If you are going to cut your hair off, then feel like you have to walk around with a hat on your head, or a scarf, or anything else in an attempt to hide it, unless you plan on wearing weaves or wigs the entire time, you shouldn't cut off your hair. You have to wear your new style with confidence, and know inside and out that you are beautiful, regardless of how much hair you have on your head. That is what makes it so liberating. You have to be confident in yourself, and know that you look good. Honestly, the same goes for your natural hair. You have to, at some point, embrace your hair. It may not be in the beginning, mine wasn't. But that is the only way you will feel good about it, and others will in turn feel good about it too. Wear your hair! Style it, twist it, curl it, wave it, braid it – embrace it.

If you are not ready to wear your hair, then DON'T. Everyone has to go at their own pace, and there is absolutely nothing wrong with that at all. I transitioned for 6 months before I did my big chop. Some people choose to do the big chop in the very beginning, and then wear wigs until their hair reached a certain length. Once again, this is all fine. You need to do what is comfortable for YOU. Just make sure that you are actually caring for the hair while it is underneath. Moisture, regular washing, regular deep conditioning, etc., are crucial factors to healthy hair. Please don't neglect the hair just because it is short, and out of sight.

Cutting your hair also has the benefit of never going through the transition phase, which can be very trying on a person, because your hair is really not meant to have two different textures at the same time. The hair takes longer to grow out, and your change to a natural lifestyle actually takes longer if you choose to transition, versus cutting the relaxed hair off.

There are some cons to cutting off your hair. There's a point while it's growing when it reaches a weird phase where it may feel like it's too short to style in familiar styles, yet too long to just leave alone. This is the time when you will have to get creative and do research; there are many styles out there for this stage that look very beautiful. Embrace hair accessories, experiment with earrings and other jewelry, and always make sure that you are put together, so your feminine beauty is always apparent and shining through.

Getting Down To Business: Surviving the Transitioning Phase

For those of you that don't start your natural journey with a Big Chop, getting through the transitioning phase can arguably be the most difficult phase of going natural. The hair can be hard to style and comb; the relaxed hair can be drier, weaker, and brittle, while the new growth appears to be out of control. The discouragement and frustration you feel during this time is enough to make many people quit along the way. I personally was so frustrated, I didn't know what to do; but just a little knowledge and support was enough to make me stick with it. Hopefully, a little information can make your transition much easier, quicker and less frustrating.

First off, let me start with the fact that everyone has to do what is comfortable for them. I chose to transition, and was very comfortable with my decision. I was not as educated as I am now about my hair, and I was very nervous and unsure about what lay ahead of me. All I knew at the time was that I was sick of the chemicals. I once read on a natural-haired website as I was trying to educate myself that people who choose to transition instead of doing the 'BC' (Big Chop) are cowards. This was a statement the website was making, not someone that was visiting. I was so offended by that! First of all, everyone has to make this life decision at their own pace. The fact that we're all on the same path is what counts. We are supposed to be encouraging each other, and nothing in that statement is encouraging. This is your hair, on *your* head, that you have to walk around with and feel comfortable. So please, take WHATEVER pace you feel at ease with, and go from there. We will all get to the goal in the end.

When my new growth was first growing out, my hair was so hard to comb, dry, and coarse that I truly believed I had mistreated my hair for so long, I permanently destroyed it and there was nothing I could do. I began to feel like because of what I'd done to it for so many years, the hair I had as a child was gone, and unless I wanted to deal with this, my only option was to go back to relaxed hair. I LITERALLY COULD NOT COMB MY HAIR. Besides breaking two combs while trying to comb it (literally), my natural hair was so much thicker and stronger than the relaxed hair that when I did get a comb through it, the relaxed hair would break right off in big clumps. No matter what I would put in my hair, my hair was dry. When I tried to put even more product in it, the product would literally sit on top of my hair and leave it greasy or oily, while my hair was STILL dry on the inside and felt wiry. Unreal. I reached a point where I would not try to comb it anymore, I would just wet it a little, use some gel and brush the outer layers of it so I could get it in one ponytail, and leave it in a bun. It looked halfway decent when it was still wet, but once it dried? That was an entirely different story. But since I didn't know what else to do, I wore this hairstyle for quite some time. My hair never looked this bad when it was relaxed, was I making a mistake?? I began to reason with myself, "Maybe I just shouldn't relax it as much. Maybe I should get a texturizer. Maybe I should get it pressed?"

One of the most important things I could hear when I was transitioning was the fact that just about everyone goes through some degree of difficulty as I did. One day, I was going through the hair store and my phone rang. It was a very close friend of the family, she lives in another state. She had beautiful, long natural hair. She mentioned something about being natural, and I told her I had been transitioning for a few months now. She was ecstatic, until I mentioned that I didn't think I could deal with it anymore because of all I mentioned above. To which she replied, "Yes I know, I went through that too. But it does pass." "WHAT? YOU?" Her hair was so beautiful. It was long and curly, and looked so soft and healthy! I thought to myself, she has "good hair," she doesn't know what the hell I'm going through (Ha! I can laugh about it now). Then I saw the pictures she took when she was transitioning. Sure enough, the natural hair growing out looked just as dry, coarse, and hard to handle as mine. There was nothing she could do to it (that she knew of at the time), so she left it in very loose buns, with the really thick matted hair at the roots, and the remaining permed hair on the ends. I was amazed. So she had to get educated on how to care for her hair too, and it didn't just magically grow out of her head that way. It was the ONE thing that kept me going. Every time I was tempted to relax it, I thought about her. This will PASS, and my hair will get better. I just needed to learn how to properly care for it, because obviously I didn't have a clue. So I stuck it out, and I learned. I read, I watched videos, I experimented, I bought different products; most of all, I left my hair alone, mostly with braids. Finally, I reached the point where I just wanted to cut the permed hair off. Even though it was still pretty short, I had a lot more information, and I was ready to try to care for it better. I can honestly say that after cutting it, it was like night and day. The hair was softer, it was manageable, I was able to comb it, and it wasn't dry. Then, over the course the next year, I went from tolerating my hair, to accepting my hair, to embracing my hair, to absolutely loving my hair! Now, I wouldn't perm it if you paid me.

The first thing you have to realize is natural hair and relaxed hair living on the same hair strand is bound to cause problems. Natural hair thrives on moisture, permed hair does not – as a matter of fact, as a rule, you try to stay away from moisture as much as possible when you have a relaxer or a fresh press. Therefore, the hair coming out of your scalp, currently attached to the relaxed hair, is literally STARVING for moisture. It's dry and feels coarse because it has no moisture (water) and it's porous (can't retain the moisture you put in it). Next, the types of products you're used to using is not meant to care for natural hair, another strike – so the moisture and nutrients it's starving for, it doesn't receive. Finally, your relaxed hair is considerably weaker than the natural hair, so with improper treatment, breakage is inevitable.

So what can you do to make your transition better than mine?

The first thing is to find, and exude, patience. Knowing what you're in for makes it easier to deal with. The next thing to do is to start treating your hair as if you're already completely natural, to fortify your new growth with all the things it's presently lacking:

- Moisturize your hair often (WATER).

- Detangle your hair in sections, just as you would when detangling a full head of natural hair, and use a wider-toothed comb (See Combing and Brushing section).

- Do not wash your hair with sulfate shampoos (this includes many over-the-counter shampoos, even expensive ones) and wash and condition your hair more often (see Shampooing section). Some even take the extra step of co-washing their hair in between hair washes to provide more moisture (see Shampooing section for more info on co-washes).

- Use VERY LITTLE or no heat during this delicate phase.

- Braids and twists are your friend – they allow your hair to stay detangled and moist, while the braids or twists pull your natural hair a little straighter and bend the relaxed hair a little curlier; allowing the hair to blend and look more uniform. Make 6-8 eight sections, delicately comb out the hair, and braid or two-strand twist the hair section by section before going to bed. Never go to bed with your hair loose: always braid, twist, or Bantu knot your hair at night, keeping the ends in and the hair moist and untangled. As your hair gets longer and you have more new growth to deal with, depending on your hair type, you may want to use more braids.

- Your hair's PH balance is most important during this phase because the hair is in a confusing state; you can consider acidic rinses to help balance the PH during this delicate phase (see PH Balance section).

- You should be washing your hair every week to 10 days and Deep Conditioning it for at least 30-40 minutes EVERY SINGLE TIME.

- Consider wearing protective styles most of the time during this stage.

This is a frustrating stage, but I have seen many make the transition so beautifully and seamlessly. Also, once you reach the point where you are comfortable with cutting off the remainder of the relaxed hair, the change in your hair should be immediate, and considerable. It should feel softer, more manageable, and easier to detangle and retain moisture. From there, with the proper care, it will only get better and better. It will be well worth the wait!

Getting Down To Business: Dreads and Sister Locks

Most people already know what dreadlocks are: Locks of hair that matt together (or "lock") to form coiled locks throughout the head. This locked hair is not combed, but many do still groom their locks (preferred). Depending on your preference, you can start dreads through many methods, including the backcombing method (teasing the hair upward towards the scalp so it can knot together); the neglect method (where you do absolutely nothing and let the hair matt on its own); or you can do the twist method, the most popular and well-groomed method for dreadlocks. It is helpful when using this method to use a locking wax or something that will aid in keeping the hair twisted, so it gets the opportunity to lock over time. One thing I will recommend is not to make the sections of locks too small, as the weight of the hair and repeated twisting over time can put too much stress on the hair and cause the hair to break, and even cause the lock to pop off. The same can be said for allowing someone to pull your new growth too tight when locking your new growth. Wearing too many tight styles (like any natural hair style) is not good for the overall health of the hair and can cause too much stress on the scalp, causing the hair to break or even pull out from the root.

Regular washing and conditioning is also necessary; some are under the impression that dreads aren't clean, and this simply isn't true. It all depends on the person, and their regimen. Others believe you shouldn't wash your dreads because it will not lock; this is not the case, and unhealthy for any scalp. Like regular natural hair, because dreads are a natural hairstyle, natural products work best.

Some hesitate to do dreads because they feel it will limit the styles they can do. This is also untrue. There are almost as many styles you can do with your dreads as you can with your regular hair: Your locks can be curled, cut, dyed, pinned up, and even braided. Then there are twist outs, braid outs, Bantu knots, ponytails; you can wear clips and other hair accessories – in short, you are not without beautiful options for your dreads. One thing: you cannot take out dreads. Once the hair locks, you will have to cut your hair off to about 2 inches if you no longer want to wear them. I have heard that some have been able to take them out with a pin, but this option is definitely not for everyone. My personal belief is this option may depend on how well your hair locked in the first place. Just know when you start that this is a huge decision, as you will more than likely have to cut it off to make a change.

Sisterlocks are similar to dreads, but with much smaller locks. Unlike dreads, you should go to a professional to start sister locks, because there are different sizes of locks in different areas of your head, and a different method used to form the locks. Because the locks are so thin, there is no wax or gels used, like traditional locks. You can also begin sisterlocks without cutting off all of your relaxed hair before starting, and gradually cut the relaxed hair as the natural hair is growing. They are meant to be a more versatile option to traditional dreads; since the hair is sectioned in much smaller pieces, it is believed that you would have many more options to style sisterlocks; though many women with dreads will certainly disagree. The downside that some complain about when starting sisterlocks is, because the hair is parted so thin, much of the scalp looks exposed, even with thick hair. According to hairdressers that do sisterlocks, this goes away slowly as your hair grows out.

Like dreads, this is not something you can just remove from your hair without cutting it all off (some say you can, but it would be a grueling process), so please be mentally prepared for this type of decision. Please visit their official website, sisterlocks.com, for more information on this hair/lifestyle choice.

Caring For Your Natural Hair: Expectations, Hair Growth, and Hair Don'ts

So there are obvious variations in our hair care versus other races that most black women already know about, otherwise we wouldn't have practically any hair on our heads at all, right? The two most obvious that most people know about is:

Wearing a scarf at night (or the cloth on your pillowcase and sheets will snag and pull at your hair, and the friction can break your hair off).

And

Less frequency in washing your hair. We can't wash our hair every day or it would be dry, brittle and break off, whereas if other races didn't wash their hair, it would look horrible because of build-up.

These are all good variances in our hair to know, and the most obvious ones. But the truth is, in order to care for our hair the correct way, the entire way we care for our hair would have to change: from the way we wash our hair, condition our hair, even DRY our hair; to what we put in our hair, the way we moisturize our hair, the way we protect our hair, the way we comb and brush our hair, and the way we prepare our hair for bed. All of these things would have to change if you want your hair to reach its full potential.

Although we've had our hair our entire lives, because we've been taught that straighter and smoother is better, many of us have done everything we can to alter our natural hair to become what society has defined as being beautiful. In doing so, we've basically been going totally against the basic structure and needs of our natural hair: with relaxers, pressing, curling irons, excessive blow-drying and heat, wash and sets, even basic hair care regimens and what we know as everyday products like crèmes, greases, and shampoos. Essentially, our hair has been suffering because it is literally starving for the basic nutrients and everyday care that our type of hair needs to thrive.

This is why when we have a touch of new growth, that hair that we see growing out appears to be what we think our natural hair essentially is and all it can be: hard to comb, dry, difficult to take in moisture, difficult to lie down, constantly breaking, and feeling coarse and wiry. This is also the reason why our black hair never seems to reach a growth that's past our shoulders.

The real truth is that many, many black women have NO IDEA what their natural hair is capable of looking or feeling like. Not the new growth from a perm; that hair is suffering from being on the same strand with a chemical relaxer and is being sucked dry and coarse from the chemicals. Not even the hair that you had before a perm when you were little, and your mom used to grease your hair with a heavy greasy product (I can still remember the smell of Dax), even though that was still a much closer version to your hair's potential before the harsh chemicals. No, I mean your hair's actual potential. Most people don't even know what their curl or coil pattern is, because they've never even seen it. Can you imagine? Having something on your head all your life and still not even knowing what it's supposed to look or feel like?

I for one would want to reach in and know my own hair's full potential, and love myself for who I am. Then if I want to change it – at least I know what I'm changing.

Results and Expectations: Like most things in the world, we live in a society that wants things in the 'now.' Unfortunately, much like weight loss, your hair didn't get like this in a day, so please don't have the false expectation that it will revert back to bouncy and healthy in a day either. I can say that once you start implementing the appropriate hair care, it should start to feel better (to the touch) in a short amount of time (it can be practically immediate). When you start putting the right products in your hair and change your way of combing and shampooing, that change can happen rather quickly. It's like your hair was starving for it all along. Depending on your present condition, the hair retention can be pretty fast as well. Within weeks, your hair should feel stronger with the right care. In a little longer time, it should be more elastic, and less prone to breakage.

It should feel less coarse to the touch, and it should begin to make changes from the inside out as the months go by. As far as your actual curl pattern, I can't say how long it will take you, but I can say that after about 8 months of care, braiding my hair and leaving it alone after my big chop, curls (that I never knew I had) were suddenly appearing. So it took my hair 8 months after braiding it and moisturizing to see my true hair pattern. I did not have all the factors in the equation of my hair care yet though, and I believe this was the reason it took my hair so long; as I have been taking care of other individuals' hair since they've gone natural and within a month, I see a huge difference.

Also, know that you cannot change your hair type, nor can you always use the same methods other naturals use to achieve the same results; you have to learn what your hair needs to achieve the results you're looking for. Starting with getting advice from women who have a similar hair type to yours is a good place to start. Be realistic about your expectations – you can achieve a similar look, but it may take a different approach or different products.

Hair Growth: Many people come up to me and ask, "How can I get my hair to grow like yours?" Some black women are under the impression that their hair only grows to their shoulders, or to their chin, etc. This is not true. I know for some, this will be hard to grasp, but it is a fact: your hair is already growing. Our hair grows just like every other race's hair. The average person's hair grows about a half an inch per month. How often did you have to get a touch up with a relaxer? For some, it's 6 weeks. For some, it's even a month. For some, they think they're "lucky" enough to only need a perm every 2 months. The more often you need a relaxer, the faster your hair grows. Hair growth is NOT the black woman's problem. The problem is actually retaining the growth that takes place in your hair. So let's examine this. Have you ever seen the remnants of when a black woman combs her hair? For many, you see short pieces of hair in the comb or on the floor. We have grown to accept this as normal, and only get concerned when it's more than usual. Now, think of when a Caucasian person combs their hair, or an

Indian person, or any other race. Hair comes out as well, but is it short little pieces? Unless their hair is breaking, the answer is no. What they leave behind is long pieces of hair in their comb. Why? Because their hair is naturally shedding, like every person's hair should, while the black woman's hair is actually breaking off. The sad fact is, as fast as our hair is growing, if the hair is over-processed, not cared for properly, or sometimes just chemically altered, oftentimes the black woman's hair is breaking off at the same rate it is growing. If you can see your hair growing, it's breaking off at a slower pace than it's growing. If you can see your hair falling out, however, then the opposite is happening.

Some people ask about hair growth phases. This is true, the hair does have a growth cycle, and that cycle has three phases: the anagen (growth) phase, the catagen (transition) phase, and the telogen (resting/shedding) phase. The key thing to know about these phases is that they all happen at the same time, with the majority of your hair in the growth phase. This is why you never know which phase is happening, or when. One strand of your hair may be in the growth phase, while the other strand's shedding, while yet another strand is resting. So you really need not be concerned with the growth phases of your hair, as they have no bearing on your hair care. Just let nature take its course. This book is not going to teach you how to grow your hair. That's not my job. Nature and your body already do that. This book is meant to teach you how to retain your hair growth, so that it can reach lengths it's never been able to reach before now. It's meant to teach you how to care for your hair so it stays healthy, feels soft, is moist from the inside out, has elasticity, is defined, and is manageable.

So what are the main components of healthy hair for maximum hair growth?

Moisture – within your hair shaft, in its cortex.

Porosity – your hair's ability to actually retain the moisture it takes in.

And elasticity – your hair's ability to stretch out longer than its normal length when pulled, and revert back without breaking or snapping off.

This book will go into great lengths about what is needed to care for your hair and obtain these components while in its natural state (they actually almost intertwine with each other, in my opinion), but let me just take a moment to generally discuss what we shouldn't do. If we're going to take the time to care for our hair, there are little things we may tend to do on a regular basis that can combat all of our efforts and make our hard work futile:

- We shouldn't use the same hair care products we used in our relaxed hair in our new natural hair. Remember, our natural hair has needs that are almost totally opposite to the needs of relaxed hair, with the most important of these factors being moisture. How could we possibly use the same products on our natural hair to do the exact opposite of what they were made for?

- Our hair should never remain in a dry state for long periods of time, and in turn become brittle.

- We shouldn't comb or brush our hair too often or vigorously. (A rule of thumb is how long it takes you to comb your hair. If it's a quick process, then you are being too vigorous with your hair, because a thick head of curly strands takes time to comb gently.)

- We should shy away from chemicals (of any kind, for any reason).

- We shouldn't leave our hair out all the time. Our hair does better when it's in protective styles.

- We shouldn't do styles in our hair that inflict unnecessary pulling of the hair and trauma to our scalp on a regular basis (tight buns, tight or tiny braids, twists or locks, tight hair-pinned styles, etc.)

- We shouldn't use our nails to scratch our scalp aggressively (it damages our cuticles).

- And finally, we shouldn't have our hands in our hair all of the time (some of us have our hands in our hair all day, what some refer to in the Natural Community as the "hands disease").

Caring For Your Natural Hair: First Things First - MOISTURIZE

If there's nothing else you take away with you after reading this book, you should learn that our hair, especially in its natural state, needs to be moisturized. This is something that many have been most confused and misled about, so let me break it down in the simplest way: The ONLY thing that can moisturize your hair is water. Let me say it again. ONLY WATER. Not crèmes, oils, or butters. WATER. Every single person with natural hair should be moisturizing their hair with water. Does this mean that you should wet your hair under a faucet or a shower every day? No. But if you're natural, you should own a small spray bottle that emits a fine mist so that your hair can get the moisture that it needs. Black women have been taught for so many years to stay away from water. We don't want our hair to frizz, curl up, or come out of a fresh press or a curl. But our hair NEEDS water to flourish properly. When you look at a natural-haired person whose curls look defined and her hair is shiny and the color pops, that is someone who moisturizes her hair. When you look at a natural-haired person whose hair looks frizzy, dry, brittle, and the ends are breaking, this is someone who is either having trouble with the PH balance and porosity of their hair (we'll discuss later), or someone who more than likely is not moisturizing their hair and locking in the moisture. Plain and simple.

Finding the right balance with moisture can be a small task in the beginning. If you wet your hair too much, it will air dry and end up really dry, much like when you wash your hair. If you don't wet it enough, however, it won't be moist enough. The goal is to lightly mist it just enough to where it maintains that moisture. For me, I find that a small spray bottle set to mist is perfect. Your hair should feel moist, but not wet. It should feel drier than what it feels like after a towel squeeze after a hair wash, but wetter than normal. You should not wet your hair with a spray bottle set to a concentrated stream, or to where your hair is dripping. It should be a mist that has a very wide aim, so all of your hair gets a small amount.

Finding what frequency works for you is mere trial and error, and can also depend on where you live (hair typically retains more moisture in humid places, and less moisture in drier places) and on your own hair type. I have thick, dense, mostly 3C hair, and although I live in a humid place, I spray my hair every single day. That works for me. Some do it every other day. Depending on your own hair type and texture, you can find out in a short time of experimenting what the right amount and frequency is for you.

Caring For Your Natural Hair: Combing and Brushing

Combing your hair would seem like the most basic thing you can do, right? I mean you've been doing it practically your whole life. Unfortunately, the fact is, one of the biggest mistakes we make is the manner in which we comb and brush our hair.

Combing and Brushing: If you have thick hair with an abundance of curls on your head and use a small, fine-toothed or rat-tailed comb to comb your hair, throw it away. You are damaging and pulling out your hair every single time you use it. Our thick, curly strands require a much wider-toothed comb. This is ALL the time, not sometimes. When combing, try not to comb all of your hair at once, but rather in sections (minimum of four). When combing and encountering a knot, gently remove the comb or brush and slowly work your way out of the knot. You can even use your hands to help detangle it before trying to comb through it again. Please don't just comb through the knot and break off your hair. Some of us are way too harsh with our hair. For regular brushing, you should always use one that has boar bristles. They are the best kind of brushes for your hair and are gentle on natural hair, unlike some other materials.

Detangling: When detangling hair, the best way to detangle your hair is when it is wet. Generally speaking, if you have natural black hair, you should never try to detangle, or even comb your hair when it is completely dry. As instructed before, you can use your spray bottle to cover your hair with a fine mist before combing. Since I mist my hair every day, I do in fact follow that method of never combing my hair completely dry. But when detangling, I actually take an extra step, and it is one that is especially advised for people with fragile, damaged, or extra-curly hair: I detangle my hair when it has conditioner in it. It gives my hair maximum slippage (ability for the hair to "slide" through the comb), and the knots are easier to detangle, leaving you with minimal damage to your hair. This works wonders for me. Whatever method you prefer, you should not try to detangle all of your hair at once. Part the hair in sections (again, minimum of four, but depending on your length or thickness, as many as you need), detangle, put the detangled hair section up (section it off), and go on to the next section. Repeat this method until the entire hair is detangled. Depending on how long your hair is, a suggestion would be to detangle your hair from the ends and work your way up to the roots; detangling the hair from the ends upward helps to reduce knots that are difficult to get out. When you encounter a knot, don't pull and force the comb or brush through – essentially breaking your hair – instead, remove the comb/brush, take your time, and slowly work through and detangle the knot. Coming in from a different direction (like the bottom) helps a great deal as well, when trying to work out a stubborn knot.

This is something that definitely requires a great deal patience at first. When I first started doing this, it was very new for me to sit there and take that much time (at least it seemed that way) to simply comb my hair. Something that I have been doing most of my life seemed like a whole new drawn-out process for me. Now, I don't even think about it. I have such a rhythm going with it now that it feels perfectly normal, and it really doesn't seem to take that much time at all. But it takes time to get there. Please be patient.

I don't have a lot of personal experience with a Denman brush, but I know many Natural women that swear by it. My sister recently tried it, and loves it for detangling her hair. I personally use a wide paddle brush (with balls on the tips). It's gentle on my hair, and if I encounter a knot, the brush has room to "give" because of the soft base, so that my hair doesn't break. Some say that the paddle brushes with balls on the tips grab onto the hair and pull it out. For as long as I have been natural, I have never encountered this. And I actually don't like the harshness of the pointy bristles of the Denman (my scalp is tender), or the amount of hair that comes out when using it, so I use what works for me. Some people 'modify' their Denman brush by removing every other row of bristles. This may work for you as well. I have recently heard of a product called the Tangle Teezer, and have read and heard some great reviews on the product. The general consensus is it greatly reduces the amount of hair that comes out when detangling.

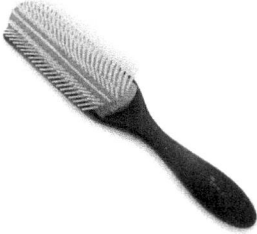
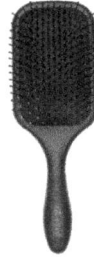

Denman Brush   Paddle Brush

Frequency: I found one constant while doing research: most women who are natural that have healthy, long hair, do not comb their hair every day. They wear their hair in styles that don't require having to comb their hair every single day, and when they wash their hair, they comb and detangle their hair to get rid of all of the hair that naturally sheds from their head. This shedded hair is not pieces of broken hair, but entire strands that come out from the root. When you start seeing full strands as opposed to pieces of hair while combing, you know that your hair is headed in the right direction. Even if you don't use the method of combing your hair every few days (which hardly anyone uses ALL the time), you should get into the practice of doing your hair and leaving it alone. You don't want to continually be combing your hair all day, or even every day.

As mentioned previously, some people use a comb to detangle, some use a Denman brush, some use a Tangle Teezer, and others use a paddle brush. There are some who will even tell you that the best comb is your human comb – your fingers. I do use my fingers to help detangle my strands when my hair is really tangled, but I still feel the need to comb it. I think you should use, and do, what is comfortable for you.

Shedding: One more important thing: Please don't freak out when you see hair coming out that has shedded from your head. This is something that I also had to get used to. A healthy head of hair can shed up to 100 hairs per day. I found it hard to believe as well, but it's a fact. And to make it worse on your mind, when you don't comb your hair on a daily basis and you finally wash and detangle your hair, or if you've had your hair in braids for an extended period of time, when you finally comb it, you will now see an accumulation of shedded hair that has been sitting in your head and is now coming out all together. This is nothing to be concerned about. It is a natural shedding process, and is perfectly normal. Hair that is naturally shedding from your head will be an entire strand of hair with the bulb; NOT pieces of broken hair coming out of your head. An entire hair strand with the bulb = natural. Shorter pieces of hair without the bulb = NOT natural = breakage.

Bonus tip: Avocado Conditioner for your hair

The same good fats in avocado that's good for your body, are also very nourishing for your hair. It will leave your hair with immediate results: soft, moisturized and smooth:

– Mash a ripe avocado in a bowl until it has a thick, soft consistency with no lumps

– Add three tbsps of Aloe Vera Gel

– Add two tbsps of Olive Oil

– Add one squeeze of your usual conditioner (optional. if not, use one tbsp of honey)

Mix together thoroughly and apply to your hair in sections like a mask, for maximum coverage. Leave on for 20–40 minutes, then thoroughly rinse out with lukewarm water. Your final rinse should be cooler than room temperature, to help close your pores and cuticles.

Caring for Your Natural Hair: Shampooing and Conditioning Your Hair

People with natural hair, just like people with relaxed hair, have varying opinions on shampoos and conditioners. I will not try to sway you, nor will I endorse any particular product, but I will say that the regular shampoos that you are used to using in your relaxed hair, just like the regular products, will generally not always do well with natural hair. I personally go to a health food supermarket and buy shampoo and conditioner that are derived from organic, natural products. You can go to a place like this, or a health food store, and buy shampoos from there. I'm sorry, but unfortunately, unless you're lucky enough to have a local grocery store that sells these types of products, this is your best bet. They can be more expensive than regular shampoos, but since you aren't spending money on relaxers, wash and sets, and touchups at the salon, you should not feel the pinch. A good middle ground is Organix, because it doesn't have sulfate or parabins in it, and you can get it in Walmart and some supermarkets.

Types of Shampoos and Conditioners: Most over-the-counter shampoos have way too many products in them that are not good for your hair. One of these products in particular is sodium laureth sulfate, or sodium lauryl ether sulfate (SLES or SLS). This ingredient is a very cheap foaming agent (the thing that causes lather) found in most shampoos (even expensive ones and baby shampoo) and even sometimes in soap and toothpaste. Most people associate foaming and lots of suds and bubbles with real cleaning power. Problem is this belief is untrue, and this product is not good for your hair. Many websites state that it can cause cancer, and a host of other diseases and ailments. I do not have enough expertise to make these types of claims. What I can tell you is what scientists say about it: besides being a severe eye and skin irritant (even in low doses), it not only strips the hair of healthy oils and damages it, leaving it split, and "fuzzy," but it also leaves deposits in your scalp and surface of your skin; which, over time, can lead to damaging your hair follicles. Scary, right? Unfortunately, like with other businesses, it's all about the buck.

Natural shampoos actually don't suds up like what you're used to. They're meant to clean your hair, not make bubbles. Please try to wrap your head around the fact that there is a difference. You will see the fact that it is cleaning, and it will suds up a bit, just not as much.

New Technique: As soon as your hair gets long enough to do this, don't wash your hair loose anymore. We have learned to wash our hair by piling it on our head and rubbing very vigorously. This is very abusive to the hair, scalp, and causes a great deal of tangling in curly tresses that now have to be detangled – causing more knots and increasing the chances of hair loss with excessive combing. Instead, try a new approach: Braid your hair in sections, about 8 very loose braids, so you can get in between the sections. The braids assure that you are as gentle to your hair as possible, you eliminate the vigorous rubbing, and you greatly decrease the chances of tangles and knots. Now you're ready to wash. Start with your scalp. Wet your hair thoroughly with warm water (not hot). Here's a small tip that I do: I actually have two shampoo bottles: one with the concentrated shampoo I buy from the store, and one with shampoo that I've diluted with water. I find it easier to work the shampoo in my hair when it's already diluted with water. Use all of the tips of your fingers (NOT your nails – this removes cuticle layers and damages your hair and scalp) and thoroughly clean your scalp. Now we can get to the hair. As I've said, most of us have been taught to wash our hair vigorously, rinse and repeat. Some even wash it a third time. The fact is, people of color, especially with natural hair, should not wash their hair repeatedly, or wash it until it feels "squeaky clean." By the time your hair feels like that, all of the natural oils in your hair have been stripped away, and that is not a healthy hair condition. Remember, it's harder for sebum to travel down our hair shaft with all of our curls; our objective when washing our hair is to wash our scalp clean of buildup and old products, and to do the same for our hair. This only requires ONE wash. Some natural people only wash their scalp, and let the shampoo already in the scalp take care of washing the hair while rinsing. I do not personally do this, but it is worth mentioning for you to know all your options. I take a sponge (I have a Sea Sponge; they're oval-shaped, beige in color, and have big holes), and wash each braid thoroughly. Then I rinse the hair still in braids by squeezing (not wringing) the hair in my fist close to the scalp so the soap can rinse out of it. Some people leave the hair hanging and squeeze the braids two or three at a time to rinse them out. I never take my hands and rub my hair or scalp vigorously; everything you do with your hair should be with gentle hands.

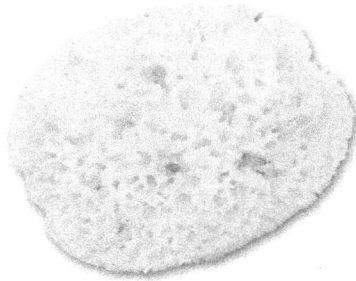

Sea Sponge

After rinsing, I towel dry my hair so it isn't dripping by holding the hair in the towel and squeezing. I NEVER take the towel and vigorously rub against my scalp, it's damaging to your hair, snags and pulls at the strands, and causes the hair to split and break. Then I begin to apply my conditioner mix. The reason I say "mix" is because my conditioner is always mixed with things. Whether it's olive oil, aloe, jojoba oil, honey, rosemary, avocado, or even a little bit of all of these things – it's usually something. I rarely just put store-bought conditioner in my hair. But this is simply a personal preference, and because all of our hair is different, doing what works best for you is the best way to go. If you want healthy hair, you MUST deep condition your hair. You must, you must, YOU MUST. Once again, a time-consuming step, but one that our hair needs. Conditioning your hair with the conditioner of your choice and putting on a cap for 20-40 minutes is a practice you should definitely get used to. While in the transition phase, I conditioned my hair for at least an hour. The only time I saw breakage in my hair (little ends in the comb and the sink) since I've been taking care of my hair properly was one week after I said to myself, "I don't have time for this today. I'll just put the conditioner in, rinse it out, and really condition it next week." Needless to say, after seeing bits of my hair in the sink that I had worked so hard to take care of, I learned my lesson. That was the last time I did that!

I condition my hair in the same sections from washing, because I also detangle my hair at this time. I loosen out (or take down) a braid, and apply the conditioner with an applicator brush (like what you use to apply a relaxer) because it is easier for me to evenly apply the conditioner to all of my hair (otherwise I'll put too much with my hands in the beginning and run out early). I work the conditioner on the entire hair shaft. Then I pay special attention to the ends. After I'm sure that the section I'm working on is thoroughly covered, I detangle by using a paddle brush and combing through the ends, working my way up the hair shaft until it's all detangled. This is when you should see your hair going through its natural hair-shedding process. Once it's fully untangled, instead of rebraiding it, I put it in a loose, two-strand twist and clip it to the side. Then I move on to the next section. I do this to my entire hair and when finished, I put on a cap. Because you are detangling while conditioner is in your hair, this can be quite a messy process! I wash my hair on Saturday mornings, and condition my hair in front of my sink with a mirror. Some do it while in the shower and confine the mess to that area, but that is not comfortable for me. I don't want to slip with all the conditioner accumulating on the floor in the shower, nor do I want to stand cold and naked for an extended period of time doing my hair. Some people buy a rubber mat for their shower/tub to prevent slipping. I clean my bathroom on Saturdays anyway, so while I have my cap on, I work up a sweat and clean up my bathroom, among other rooms in the house; which makes the conditioner penetrate my hair and leaves my hair really soft. Please do whatever works for you.

After rinsing out the conditioner, once again towel squeeze your hair (using the method mentioned above). Now you are ready to apply a leave-in conditioning product of your choice to your hair. (We will discuss this in the very next section). Once you have done that, a suggestion is to either braid your hair or twist your hair so that it can air-dry while in a protective style, and so that it is in a semi-taut (stretched) state while drying. This makes it easier to handle and style. I do not use heat to dry my hair; I allow it to dry naturally.

Co-Washing: Many naturals co-wash, and absolutely rave about its results. Co-washing is short for conditioner washing. It basically means that instead of using shampoo to wash your hair, you use conditioner to wash it. Many do this because of the fact that sulfates in shampoo can strip your hair, or the belief that shampoo can rid your hair of its natural oils (which, in fact, can be true if you're using most over-the-counter shampoos). They also believe that their hair can stay moisturized longer using this co-washing method. The idea of co-washing has actually spread beyond women of color, and other races and women with other hair textures are now co-washing as well, even if it's just in between shampoo washes to add some relief to the drying effect shampooing can have. If you decide to give co-washing a try, please make sure not to use a conditioner that has silicone in it, because you want something that will leave as little deposit on your hair as possible. There's no need to buy anything too expensive, but you should pay attention to the condition of your hair while making this transition to make sure you are not gradually forming build-up in your hair. For those that use a lot of gels and sprays in their hair, or if your hair is just naturally oily, your hair may require something stronger than conditioner to clean out the residual products or oils that are in your hair, and co-washing may not necessarily be the right regimen for you.

Frequency: Most of us have been taught that we cannot wash our hair as often as other cultures because of the drying affect it can have on our hair, and this is true. But does that mean that we should wash our hair once every 2, or even 3 weeks? The fact is, in order for the hair to be in a healthy state and a growing environment, the scalp needs to be clean. This is just a fact, and the fact that we have drier hair doesn't change this. It is especially true that using harsh shampoos can be very drying for the hair, but if you are using a gentler, all-natural shampoo, you should have no problem being able to wash your hair every 7 to 10 days. This is the average that you should be washing your hair, and freeing your scalp of product buildup. It also stimulates the scalp when you massage it while washing. Some people wash it even more often, but this is something you should individually determine, based on your hair texture, density, and lifestyle. Washing your hair every two to three weeks, however, is just too long, and not maintaining a growing, healthy environment for your hair.

Bonus – Leave-in recipe (for thick hair, 3C–4A, to restore moisture and balance PH):

1/4 Cup of Aloe Gel (Whole Leaf)

1/8 Cup of Kinky Curly Knot Today (one good squeeze of the bottle)

2 Tbsps of Vegetable Glycerin

3 Tbsps of Olive Oil (Cold Pressed, Virgin)

1 Tbsp of Castor Oil

1 Tbsp of Jojoba oil

1 Tbsp of Coconut Oil

Mix together and apply to hair sections while it is still damp, concentrating on ends; seal hair with a little Shea butter, then twist or braid your hair and let it air-dry naturally. Put the remainder in the fridge and reapply in a few days, to keep the hair moist in between washes.

*Measurements are just an approximation; use more or less as needed/desired.

Caring For Your Natural Hair: Hair Care Products

As I briefly mentioned before, the hair care products you used in your relaxed hair will more than likely not fare well in your new natural tresses. It will possibly leave your hair very dry, and very thirsty. For me, and for many people whose hair is natural, healthy, and steadily increasing in length, we find it better to use natural products for the hair, or at least shampoos, conditioners, etc. that have more natural products in them. In this section, I will mention some store-bought products for natural hair that I am familiar with; you can take this information and do further research on each product as you see fit. I will also provide you with information on natural oils and products for your hair that you can buy yourself and mix for your own needs; once again as you see fit.

Our type of hair is determined by our genes, with each of us having our own unique mix of traits. Because of this, we all have to go through a period of trial and error until you find the right blend of products that is specific to your own hair's needs. Some may need more oil, some may need more crème, some may need more water. Some may need a larger quantity of products than others. There is no set regimen written in stone. The amount of oils, plants and natural butters that you can use in your hair are endless, but most healthy-haired people find what works for them and stick with it. Unlike the thinking many people have when their hair is relaxed, natural hair tends to like consistency, so developing a routine is a very healthy process. Find what works for you, and try to stick with it. Besides a few other elements, the actual assortment of natural oils, herbs, plants and butters that are known for promoting healthy hair is where you should start. You then just have to determine the right amount of ingredients you need of each thing (based on your hair needs), or if your hair condition needs it at all. If your hair is dry, use more products that help this condition. If your hair needs more elasticity, use oils that promote and maintain this, and so on. Before long, your hair regimen will become something you would have perfected that is just right for your own hair.

First, some bad news. There is no set product that will work for everyone. I'm sorry, but because each of us have different types and textures of hair, you will not find something that will work for every single person. You simply have to experiment and see what works for you. Knowing your hair type is a great place to start. This stage of your natural hair care experience may start with a great deal of trial and error. I had a closet full of products that I tried until I found what worked for ME. Things that people have raved about, I sometimes didn't like, and some of the brands I use, I've never heard anyone rave about; I just liked the ingredients, tried it, and loved it. But I will later give you as much of a general breakdown as I can for your hair type, just to give you a starting point.

One disclaimer: I really don't experiment with many store-bought products on my hair anymore. When I first stopped relaxing my hair and the first year after my big chop, I experimented heavily with products, trying to find what was right for me. Then, I began to grow tired of constantly reading ingredients and reasoned with myself, "If I'm buying this product for the shea butter (for example), why not just buy natural shea butter instead of worrying how much shea butter was actually in this product, along with other things I DIDN'T want in my hair?" This newfound thinking just grew into where I am today, with about 90% of all the products I use in my hair being 100% natural. I have also, along the way, found store-bought products and lines that are also fully natural and great for my hair, and have incorporated them into my regimen. The natural stuff works great for me, and I would not look back. But the added work of finding, ordering or obtaining natural products and conditioners is not for everyone, so I am just going to try to give you a point you can start from to find your own direction. Also, besides basic shampoos and conditioners, I normally only use products at this point for a certain look or definition, and one of my problems with store bought products with my natural hair (actually, even before my hair was natural) is I never like the way most of them make my hair feel. In a perfect world, I would love for my hair to look the way it does when it is wet (very defined and stretched out, so my length shows), yet feel the way it does when it's dry (soft and moisturized, but not wet). I have been trying to come out of my shell and try different products meant for natural hair. The problem is a lot of them, in order to achieve this defined look, either leave your hair with a crunchy feeling, or with a greasy, gel feeling, followed by residue and flakes in your hair. I greatly don't like either of these. I hate the gel feeling, and I despise the crunchy feeling. The only medium I'm willing to compromise with is a creamy product that leaves my hair slightly heavier than usual, but not too greasy – while still achieving defined results. I have found a few that I like. But I am still searching. So in the meantime, I do my twist outs, braid outs, and other styles that give me a defined look.

I am not endorsing any products, nor am I getting paid by anyone; I am simply letting you know of the products I've heard and read about from other natural women, and informing you of the products I use or have experimented with. Also, like store-bought hair care, you will have to find your own balance of the natural oils and butters for your own hair and its needs. I will give you a breakdown of the oils, what they are good for, and tell you if I've tried them and if they work for me. Since this is mostly what I use now as opposed to store-bought products, this section will be pretty extensive. Once again, this is all just a guide:

Store-bought products and hair care lines (in no particular order):

Organix – Organix is a line of shampoos and conditioners that promote a unique blend of natural ingredients in each line. They are sulfate and parabin free, which is great. They have a coconut milk line, as well as their mandarin olive oil, tea tree oil, shea butter, vanilla silk, cocoa butter, and cherry blossom ginseng lines, among others. I actually used Organix for about a year (my first year without a perm). I used the Coconut Milk line, and I thought it worked fine with my hair. I only stopped as I transitioned into buying 100% natural products for my hair, but I can honestly say that for someone who doesn't want to travel far for the natural stuff or doesn't want to buy natural shampoos and conditioners online, I think this is a great middle ground. Although they are not 100% natural, the lack of sulfate and addition of natural products brings this line up a considerable notch. I know someone who grew her hair way down her back and she was using Organix at the time (coconut milk line as well), so I think the potential is definitely there if you're using great products as leave-in conditioners for your hair in addition to the Organix. It has proteins in it (egg white proteins), so if your hair is sensitive to that, be careful. My hair isn't, so it worked fine for me.

APHogee – This line is something I hear a lot of naturals rave about as well. The things I've heard the most about are the Keratin Reconstructers and the protein treatments. I have never used any of them. But I have heard people, natural and otherwise, claim great results for those who have damaged hair. Note: Please see the section in this chapter regarding the use of proteins in your hair.

Miss Jessie's – Miss Jessie's has Salons in NY that cater to naturally curly hair, as well as people who have texturizers. They also have products that they sell for people who may not be in their area, and have plenty of instruction online and in brochures to achieve salon-like results. Of them, the four I'm most familiar with are the Curly Pudding, the Curly Meringue, the Stretch Silkening Crème and the Curly Buttercreme. I've used Miss Jessie's Curly Pudding once, while my hair was still in the short, curly phase. It looked great: really defined, moist and curly. Once my hair dried, however, it felt crunchy. This is a serious negative for me, as I despise that feeling in my hair. This is why I've never used hair sprays and hard gels, even when I had a relaxer. A good friend of mine, however, has a fine grade of 3A hair, and one day, when asking her about products, she told me she uses the

Curly Pudding. Her hair always looks so great and naturally defined, and it was soft. She applies the curly pudding to her dry hair and puts it in Bantu Knots at night to achieve her curly look. It looks so nice all the time that I thought it was her natural curl pattern. So it could be a great product for some, and maybe not so much for others. Or it's possible that I just applied it wrong (I won't rule that out, it was early in my natural hair process). Most Type 3s that I've talked to don't like it, but MANY Type 4s love Miss Jessie's because it gives their hair more hold and definition that will last, versus other brands. Miss Jessie's has a whole line of products catered to the naturally curly community. My opinion would be to try them for yourself to see if it works for you. They can be a bit pricey though, so keep that in mind (one local Miami hairdresser sells the big containers [like the size of a regular jar of hair gel] for about $50, but the website sells the same bottle for considerably less – $38). There are places where you can buy the smaller containers, or you can buy it online as well). They recently started selling the line in Target, but I don't know what the prices are in their stores.

Eco Styler Curling Gel – People with Type 4 hair swear by this product, so much so that I was prone to try it. This was before I was aware of what my hair type was, but even back then, I never liked gels. I can say though that it is a fairly decent product: not too greasy, a little goes a very long way, and it has a pleasant smell. I bought the kind that has aloe vera in it. Like I said, I don't like gels, so I used it only once; but when I did, it was a fairly good experience – the hair looked defined and shiny; it was just a little too heavy for my taste.

Infusium 23 – Infusium 23 Pro-Vitamin Original hair treatment is probably the only thing I used in my hair daily (long after I made the 'natural products' transition) that was not organic. I am not promoting or disparaging it, I just want to be totally honest with my experience. It is water-based, and although it is not all natural, I felt like it did the job I wanted it to, which was to help keep my hair moist while it was in the braids. It was recommended to me by another natural-haired woman that has very long hair (to the end of her back), and she swore by it when she used to wear braid extensions in her hair. I started using it right after my big chop and during that time, I also had my hair in braids all the time. As my hair grew and I transitioned to more organic products, I still couldn't find it in me to leave that behind. I'd pour it in a spray bottle and spray it in my hair each morning to help to keep my hair moist. I have heard a few other people with natural hair say the same. Some dilute it with more water – I did not, because I used my water bottle and other products in addition to my bottle with the Infusium 23.

As time went on, however, and I began to educate myself, I became more and more conscious of the products I was using in my hair that weren't natural, so I began to have more interest in what was in it. So finally one day, I begrudgingly decided to do my research on its in-gredients. I pay special attention to the ingredients that come first, be-cause ingredients are listed in order of quantity. The second thing after water was "Amodimethicone." My general rule of thumb is to stay away from products that have ingredients I can't even pronounce. As I looked further and further into the ingredients, I found that almost all of the ingredients were words I didn't know. That didn't sit well with me. Besides glycerin, castor oil, and fragrance, I couldn't tell you what the rest of the ingredients even were without an encyclopedia. So, that was the end of my relationship with Infusium 23, and honestly, my hair's condition didn't change at all, so maybe it was mental (smile). But for what it's worth, I do believe it did fine for my hair when I was using it.

African Royale – African Royale braid and extensions sheen spray is something I also discovered while my hair was in extensions. It was something I used daily with water and Infusium to help nourish my hair when it was in the braids, and I have to say, once again, although not completely natural, it worked fine. It has Propylene Glycol high on its ingredient list, which is a cosmetic form of mineral oil used for shine (but not necessarily good for your hair); but it also has many fortifying vitamins and herbs in its ingredients, including Glycerin, Silk Amino Protein, Wheat Germ, Sage, Henna, Comfrey, Burdock

Root, Goldenseal, Cherry Bark, and Chamomile, among many others. It also now has Tea Tree Oil in it to help with itching. Based on the more natural ingredients, in my opinion, it is better for your hair than the Infusium. When I took my hair out of the braids, it was so moist, soft and manageable, which was a far cry from how my hair USED to look when I took it out of braids (I don't want to frighten you all with the details, but think dry, flaky, brittle), so I thought I might pass on the information in an unbiased form – use it as you so choose.

Organic Root Stimulator – ORS has some really good products. This line, in my opinion, is also a great medium if you want to find an over-the-counter line that may not be all-natural, but still does well for your hair and is more easily accessible to purchase. I've used some products from the Olive Oil line – the Incredibly Rich Hair Lotion, and one product I really loved was the Olive Oil Smooth-n-Hold Pudding. I think they both did really well in my hair, and I still cheat on my natural products with the pudding every once in a while to give my edges a soft hold so it looks neat. My sister has used more of the line and really likes them, though she has type 4 hair and did not care for the pudding much. I don't know if this is an indication that it works better for type 3 hair than type 4, but I think it's a really nice product to give you a soft hold while keeping your edges down, especially when your hair is shorter and needs something light to help make it look a little neater.

Protein treatments – I'm just going to throw protein treatments in here because they are something that some naturals do to their hair (not all). Protein treatments can consist of keratin reconstructing conditioners, silk amino treatments, collagen protein, even wheat protein treatments. The natural protein in the hair (keratin) is insoluble (water resistant) and very strong. It is meant to protect the hair shaft, and seal in moisture. But when it is damaged – usually from extreme heat, strong chemicals, or over processing – Protein treatments are meant to repair hair and restore the protein back to normal. Many swear by them, and feel that they do a great deal to strengthen their hair and repair damage in the cuticles. Some however, intentionally stay away from them.

One problem with protein treatments is adding protein to hair that doesn't need it, or using too much protein or too often, can cause a very adverse effect. Keratin is naturally meant to strengthen and seal the hair. But if you add more keratin than needed, or for some, even use keratin that isn't naturally formed in your hair, it can actually form too many layers that weigh down the hair shaft and seal the hair to the point where it prevents moisture from coming in. This can result in dry hair, brittle hair, and hair that is very hard and stiff to the touch. This is why many will tell you to use it "sparingly."

I don't use protein treatments, but I've never had a need for them, nor do I use products or practice regular habits that would break down my natural protein. For this reason, I cannot attest to its effectiveness. As I mentioned, many swear by it, but some stay away from it like the plague, shying away from products that indicate they even have a hint of protein. I don't fall in either category. The protein treatment I hear the most positive things about is the silk amino treatments, which are generally not as strong as some of the others, and is the simplest form of protein. The best advice I can tell you is not to fix something that isn't broken. If your hair is in a healthy state, try to stray from the practice of trying everything simply because you heard about what it's done for someone else, whose hair state may be different from yours. Also, prevention and a good healthy regimen in your hair are always better than a cure for damage, so please keep that in mind.

Natural Products (or pretty darn close to it):

Carol's Daughter

Carol's daughter has a great line of natural products that do well for people who have natural hair. They can be purchased on carolsdaughter.com, and I've recently also seen them in Macys. I purchased a few things from Carol's daughter when I first started transitioning to go natural, and I had good results, especially considering the state my hair was in at that time. I purchased the hair milk, the elixir, and the hair balm. Out of all of them, I really liked the hair milk for everyday use, and the hair balm for nourishing my hair when I flat-ironed it. The hair balm is very thick, and actually goes a very long way. I know someone else who tried it on her daughter, and she said the hair milk did wonders for her child's hair.

My only problem is my hair eats up product like it's hair candy, so the hair milk finished rather quickly; and I don't like having to purchase things online that's for my everyday use (unless it's a size that can last me for months). They do have store locations, but there aren't any near me; so my only option would be Macys. In my research, I've found that Carol's daughter gets great reviews for people who have a hair type in the 2s to early 3s, or hair that is of a fine texture. The hair balm and elixir bottles, if bought together (at the time of writing this book), were at a sale price of $33, while the hair milk trio, once again with a sale, was $55.

Jane Carter Solution

Jane Carter Solution is a natural hair line that has styling products for natural hair. I will be the first to admit that I was initially taken aback by the name, and wondered what kind of products they really had and for whom (please don't judge me too harshly!). Many Type 3As and Bs love Jane Carter because their crèmes are light and don't weigh the hair down as much. Some 3Cs as well. I couldn't find too many Type 4s that cared for their products; they were not satisfied with the definition. Since their ingredients looked up to par and I was trying to get out of my shell and try new things, I decided they may be a worth a try. I bought two products: Condition and Sculpt, and Wrap and Roll. I used the Wrap and Roll one day when I was experimenting with my hair; I put my hair in 2 very large Bantu knots so I could have a stretched out look with big wavy ends (actually two ponytails, then twisted up the ends and tucked them in like Bantu knots). The results were not what I expected (my hair reverted back rather quickly) but still nice, and the curls were stretched out for the evening. The only con about this product was when I washed my hair, it had a considerable amount of buildup left on the hair and in my scalp, which was harder to wash out than usual. But that was my only down side. It didn't feel like gel, and it didn't make my hair hard, only slightly heavier. The Condition and Sculpt, I haven't tried yet, because the day I went to try it, I read the bottle and it said, "Dries crunchy." Whoa. I don't like that. I should have read the bottle before I actually purchased it. But I will try it eventually, maybe on a day before I wash my hair. They have a new curl defining crème that looks very promising. Problem is it comes in a huge tub that's $34.00. I have a problem spending that much for something that I don't know will work well in my hair yet (sorry). So we'll see what happens, maybe someone will have some and I can try it. Or we can all petition for a smaller bottle!

Hugo Naturals

Hugo Naturals boasts all-natural organic products: soaps, shampoos, conditioners, styling crèmes, and other adult as well as baby products. You can find them at many organic food supermarkets. I use a Hugo Naturals Shampoo, and I love it. They have different kinds of shampoo for normal hair, dry hair, chemically treated hair, or oily hair. I tend to use shampoos and conditioners for dry hair, not because my hair is unhealthy, but because I want my hair to get as much moisture treatment as possible. And because they're 100% natural, I don't worry about anything being too harsh. The Red Tea & Ylang-Ylang shampoo works very well for me.

Giovanni Organic Hair Care

The Giovanni line is an organic hair care line that is great for our curly strands. I use the Deeper Moisture, Smooth as Silk Conditioner and mix it with other things like olive oil, aloe and whatever else I desire at the time. I love this conditioner, and it works very well all on its own; the adding of other oils or herbs is just my preference. They have many different choices of shampoos and conditioners in their line, depending on your needs. They were also the line that gave me a natural-based heat protectant. I LOVE it. I'm a pretty consistent person with my hair, so I no longer go out and try things often that are outside of my regimen. I can't therefore give you an honest evaluation about the other products they have, but overall they are an awesome brand, and worth checking out. I find them at Whole Foods (I love Whole Foods) but if you look online, I'm sure you can find out how you can purchase them in your area.

Mixed Chicks

I stumbled upon Mixed Chicks while browsing, and decided to research it further. For some, it can be an awesome set of products. Many women, and women that have natural-haired children, don't know where to begin to define their curls because many products may be too heavy or greasy for their hair, but they still need something to help with definition, detangling, and softness. Let me first say that although two multi-racial women created this line for mixed hair, it works very well on defining particularly Type 3 hair, no matter what your ethnicity is. I've seen Type 3As all the way to 4As use this brand and get great definition. I also find that people who have several hair types in their hair love this product because it gives the hair a unified, defined look; which can be hard to do sometimes because the product you're using may be good for one hair type in your hair, and not another. Two products to try are the deep conditioner and the leave-in conditioner. Not greasy, not heavy, yet very defining. My kind of product, absolutely.

Curl Junkie

Curl Junkie is not 100% natural. BUT, they are pretty darn close to it. They use a lot of great organic products in their hair care line, and many naturals love them. One thing I like about them is fact that so many people with different hair types (and even backgrounds) have great things to say about their products. From Type 2 hair to finer Type 4 hair. Thicker Type 4s don't seem to get much out of it, but I've found that Type 4s with finer hair like them just as much as the other hair types. The products to try are the Curls in a bottle (says it's for finer hair, but some thicker-haired women like it as well) – it has good reviews: great definition and a light formula, women said one plus about this product was the minimal shrinkage; Aloe Fix – good reviews for this on wet and dry hair; and Hibiscus & Banana Honey Butta Leave-in (not a typo, that's what it's called) – women said it smells awesome, plus it's rich and creamy, and leaves the hair soft (thick-haired women especially love this product).

Burt's Bees

Burt's Bees offers "earth-friendly, natural personal care" products. The good thing about Burt's Bees is if you decide to use this brand, in my opinion, they are easier to find than many other natural lines. They have many natural shampoos, conditioners and treatments to choose from, and are supposed to be very gentle for the hair. I have actually tried a few of their products, but they were not hair products. My cousin has Type 4A hair, very fine in texture with beautiful hairpin-sized curls, and she loves them.

Taliah Waajid

I heard great things about some of Taliah Waajid's products and was very impressed when we tried them out. When doing research, because everyone's hair is different, you almost always get a mixture of positive and negative reviews. For this line, however, a vast majority had great things to say about these three products: The Protective Mist Bodifier, the Lock it Up Gel, and the Enhancing Herbal Conditioner. I heard the conditioner has amazing slippage, the Lock it Up Gel offers a more stretched out look for your twist outs without being stiff or flaky, and the Protective Mist Bodifier offers great shine and makes the hair feels very soft to the touch. I now use the Bodifier in addition to my regular regime. It smells great and leaves my hair feeling soft. My sister's hair is Type 4A, and she loves it and uses it all the time as well. She has also tried the Lock it Up Gel and also loves it, which is especially impressive to me because it's hard for her to find something to give her curls definition without it feeling hard. But it gives her the definition she wants, while leaving her hair soft and shiny. I personally recently found a new use for the Lock it Up Gel: I use it for my edges. AMAZING. Every gel that I've used in the past was usually heavy, but still starting out looking great. Then after some hours, it ended up looking and feeling greasy, and not good at all. The Lock It up Gel has a much lighter consistency than regular gels, and when I put it in my hair, it defines my waves, yet it does not leave behind a gel look at all. Then later in the day when I look at my hair, it still looks great, it doesn't look greasy, and everything is still in place. It is my new staple for my edges. In my opinion, they have some great products.

Oyin Hand Made

I have not personally used their products, but I have always heard great things about them. The biggest thing that I always hear and read about is their burnt sugar hair pomade. Women of every hair type love this product, and I always hear about how great it smells. Type 4s rave about the Honey Hemp Conditioner and how soft it makes their hair feel. The Shine and Define: I hear from 3Bs and Cs that it is absolutely great, while many Type 4s don't think it provides them with enough definition, but still think it's an ok product. The Greg Juice and Juices and Berries (both herbal leave-ins): I get very mixed reviews on both ends of the scale from all hair types, so I'm not sure what kind of hair loves these items. Some reviews are that they absolutely love them, some are that they saw and felt no difference whatsoever. Because of this, for those two, you'll have to use trial and error.

Beautiful Curls

I found Beautiful Curls entirely by accident, and what a GREAT FIND! I saw them in Whole Foods one day while looking for something else. What attracted me to them was the bottle. The Deep Conditioner was in a jar. That implied to me that it would be nice and thick, and my hair loves that type of conditioner. So I picked it up, and the ingredients were awesome, so I bought it. LOVE IT! They are made from certified fair trade Shea Butter, and also have a line that is made for babies and up (Curl Nurturing line). After trying the deep conditioner, I bought the shampoo. Besides Curl Nurturing, they have a Curl Activating line, and a Curl Enhancing line. I honestly never heard of them before my find, but I am here to tell you that they're the truth! Try them, especially if you have Type 4 hair that would love their thick, nurturing, buttery texture and ingredients.

Taiykel Afro Detangler

According to reviews concerning this product, it's great. I've never tested it myself, but I will say the natural ingredients look most promising: water, avocado/mango/shea butter, vitamin E, avocado oil, lecithin, green tea extract, orange extract, natural fragrance, and Citro-Zine™ (organic) as a preservative. I have learned of very good results for use with children's hair, as it is all-natural and is known for its benefits of effectively detangling and softening children's hair, so it is easier to comb and manage. One downside many have mentioned is the amount of time it takes to come, and the price ($49). This is for a half-gallon of product though, so that has to be taken into account as well.

Kinky Curly

Kinky Curly is a line that caters to the natural-haired folk, and they can be found online or in a Whole Foods Market if you're near one. The products most people talk about are the Curling Custard, the Spiral Spritz, and the Knot Today. Before trying these products, I watched online as someone did an unbiased review on the Curling Custard and the Spiral Spritz. After trying it, I can say she was spot on. She basically said a few key things: (a) If you don't use the Curling Custard as directed, you more than likely will not achieve desirable results; (b) The Spiral Spritz is lighter than the Custard, and meant to be used to revitalize the curls after a few days; but if you have Type 3 hair, the Spiral Spritz might be all you need to achieve the defined curls you desire.

I bought the Curling Custard and the Spiral Spritz when I was still experimenting with products. I like the smell of the Custard, but when I heard "custard," I immediately thought of something creamy. It is not. It is a clear substance that at first glance looks like gel, but has a heavier consistency than gel. It appeared too heavy for my hair at first, but one day I gathered the courage and gave a try. It looked totally fine, just felt greasy. The next day, the defined curls were still there, and since some of the product was absorbed, I actually liked my hair the better the next day because my hair didn't feel as greasy. I think it would be perfect for type 4 hair. The results I've seen for people with this hair type are really great, bouncy, non-greasy curls that stay defined, even the next day. The Spiral Spritz, however, is a much thinner gel than the custard. So much so, that it came in a spray pump bottle that sprayed out gel. Weird, right? But it was right on the mark for my hair. A little went a long way, and I had a great look when I used this product all by itself, without the greasy feeling. Only thing is you may want to use a diffuser (on warm, not hot) when using the Spritz or the Custard, because both can cause a great deal of shrinkage. Overall, both of these are good products, but I really don't use them often: You should use as directed to get the best results, and one of the general rules of thumb for this, and many other styling products, is to avoid using them with other products because they generally don't mix well. That's a problem for me because I'm not depriving my hair of aloe, shea butter, olive and coconut oil, or anything else I regularly use in my hair for ANY product, so I can't use any of these things often. I've used both the Custard and Spiral Spritz to obtain defined curls by wetting the hair then applying, and then I washed it out the following day. I just add it to whatever else is in my hair; but that's really not the directions, and can cause a white residue. In other words, don't follow me; I just do my own thing.

Now the Knot Today? I absolutely LOVE this product from Kinky Curly. Its primary ingredient is organic mango fruit extract. For my hair, it's a nourishing, yet light, non-greasy formula. I mix it in with my leave-in products, and it does great by my hair. It's hard for me to find, so when I do, I buy many bottles.

Cantu Shea Butter

Like The Kinky Curly, Cantu Shea Butter should not be used with other products, or doing this will more than likely result in flakes or white balls in your hair. I did not know this when I tried it, and it immediately went in the trash after my initial flaky experience. I have learned, however, that many people absolutely love this product, and use it after washing as a leave-in conditioner. It seems that people with thicker hair love it more than people with finer hair, and Type 4s favor it more than Type 3s. It is definitely a staple product for some, and they cannot do without it. If you are going to try it, please use it as directed.

Nairobi Wrapp-It Shine Foaming Lotion

There are two things I don't like about styling products: the gel feeling, and the crunchy feeling. I had to go back into the final edits of the book to add this product, because it has neither. I am speechless about this product. It has a great hold, but not a stiff hold. It's not crunchy, it's not heavy, and it keeps the style and helps your hair to stay stretched out. When me and the girls went to the natural hair salon to get our hair done for a photoshoot, The hairstylist used this on all the girls. We had 15 girls, ranging from 2B hair all the way to 4B hair. Before we left, WE ALL had a bottle in our hands to buy it and take this product home. My sister has 4A hair, and her biggest complaint is that she takes all this time to do her hair in a style and by the time she is ready to go out, it shrinks right back to its natural state and doesn't keep the intended style. But she was so impressed with this lotion. She was able to keep the hairstyle the beautician did for days, and when she tried another style herself with the lotion, it still worked very well. Everyone had similar stories. I highly recommend it for all hair types.

Natural Oils, Butters, and Herbs

Before getting into the different oils, plants, and butters, I first need to provide a little breakdown on the oils. There are two different types of oils: Carrier/base oils, and essential oils. Essential oils are pure oils from a plant, tree, or bark. Essential oils almost always have a distinct aroma, and each have their own therapeutic or even medicinal purpose, but are very concentrated and can sometimes be irritating to the skin or scalp if used in its potent form. Since they do not fully mix with water, carrier oils (also called base oils) are what are used to dilute the essential oils and essentially, *carry* them onto the skin or scalp.

A carrier oil is usually taken from the fatty portion of a plant; usually from seeds, nuts, or kernels. Carrier oils have their own therapeutic benefits, and are good for your hair and skin, just like essential oils.

Depending on the essential oil, it can be mixed in the carrier oil, sometimes by as little as a few drops to many tablespoons of carrier oil. Usually when you buy them, they have instructions on how you should dilute each one. Personally, I use more carrier oils in my hair on a daily basis, with the essential oils being used while conditioning or washing my hair. But it's your preference, and based on your own hair's needs. PLEASE REMEMBER that NO PRODUCT replaces water. ONLY WATER moisturizes the hair. So your best bet would be to apply a mist of water, then apply products to nourish, fortify, and SEAL the hair to lock in moisture, so it stays moist. If you do the reverse, your hair seals (cuticles close) before it has gotten chance to absorb the moisture from the water. Another option – I drop a few drops of my preferred oils to my water bottle as well; you can experiment and based on your needs, find what oils work best for you.

Olive oil – Carrier Oil: Olive oil adds a great deal of shine to the hair shaft and smoothes the cuticles so it doesn't feel coarse. It nourishes, strengthens and conditions the hair, making the color rich and the hair lustrous. Effectiveness: Out of everything I put in my hair, Olive oil is one of the staples I cannot do without. I put it in my deep conditioner, my leave-in, my shea butter mix, and even my water bottle. I think it works wonders in the hair and makes it shiny, radiant, and makes the color pop. My hair used to look dull when I first went natural, but once I began using Olive Oil, I don't have that problem anymore. Make sure the olive oil you use is VIRGIN. Other than that, the brand really doesn't make too much of a difference, in my opinion.

Coconut oil – Carrier Oil: Coconut oil has the proteins needed to fortify the hair, which makes it a great aid for unhealthy or damaged hair. It oils the hair shaft, and makes the hair feel soft to the touch. It also conditions the scalp, and helps to aid in relieving dandruff. Effectiveness: Coconut oil works great in my hair. It is also something I use very often in a lot of things. What I can actually see is that it makes my hair feel soft and silky, and it stops my scalp from being dry.

Shea Butter: Shea butter is a great product for the hair. It improves the texture of your hair, moisturizes the hair, and promotes hair growth if applied to the scalp. It helps to heal dry and brittle hair, and can also be used as a protective shield for the hair from the weather and even chlorine when swimming. Effectiveness: Another staple product for me, I use raw, unrefined shea butter in my hair. I love its moisturizing properties, and feel lost when I don't have any. When I buy the raw shea butter, it comes in a hard block in a small tub. By simply setting the tub in a bowl of hot water, the hard butter will melt into oil very quickly. I then mix it with some olive oil, coconut oil, jojoba oil, and Avocado oil if I have some. Then I let it sit overnight, and it solidifies into this very soft butter that is much easier to apply in my hair. Some people don't like the smell of raw shea butter (the smell is not strong at all, it just isn't a pleasant common "hair product smell"), so they mix it with burnt sugar pomade (mentioned earlier) that smells so good, and they love the results. Whatever you decide to mix it with, you do need to mix it with something, as the block that comes to you is pretty hard, and can prove difficult to apply to your hair unless you melt it for every single use.

Aloe Vera Gel or Juice: Aloe is truly amazing for the hair. It is known to be the most common natural remedy for hair loss, it penetrates the follicles and restores moisture to the strand and the scalp. It restores a balanced PH after a wash, and it contains 20 minerals and 7 vitamins good for the hair. It's also antibacterial, and helps to clean excess sebum from the hair, allowing the hair to grow and thrive. Wow. Like I said, AMAZING for the hair. Effectiveness: Before I found aloe, when I used to wash and condition my hair and braid it, the ends used to fray out and look fuzzy after it all dried (kind of like an old broom). Once I found aloe, my hair looks defined from the root to the very tips of my hair. The entire strand holds in its moisture, and I don't worry about my hair needing anything extra to restore its PH balance. Aloe is water-based, so the best thing to do is to mix it with essential oils to nourish and seal the hair as well. I also use the whole leaf gel instead of the juice. It's just easier to mix and apply to my hair. They're both all-natural. I personally use the brand '365 degrees.' I get it from Whole Foods.

Castor Oil – Carrier Oil: Castor oil nourishes the hair and locks in moisture, and is great at thickening hair that is thinning out. It also helps the hair to achieve and maintain elasticity and shine. Effectiveness: I love Castor oil for the elasticity benefits it gives to my hair. The elasticity that I have in my hair now, I never knew it was possible. It's what helps you retain your hair growth instead of it breaking off at the slightest tension or pulling. The littlest thing can make your hair snag. It can get caught on or inside of many things, like a hair clip or hairpin, a comb, even a chain around your neck. It can get tangled in a knot, or be pulled too tightly in a bun, or a small piece can get caught in a section of hair that it doesn't belong in while braiding or sectioning the hair off for different styles. Elasticity provides your hair with just a little 'give,' so instead of it snapping and breaking off, the hair "stretches" (like an elastic band) and snaps back, protecting you from losing it at the onset of the tension or trauma. One day I was taking my shades off and one of my hairs got caught in the shades. Without thinking, I instinctively let go because I didn't want the hair to snap off, but in doing so, the shades were now hanging from my one little hair strand. The weight of the shades was pulling on the hair and it hurt, but the hair did not break. I was so surprised at that. And it was a hair that was located right at the hairline of my hair, directly above my ear, which was even more impressive for me because until I went natural, that hair never used to grow and always remained short. Elasticity is definitely something you should strive to achieve in your hair. I think the overall health of your hair and a combination of oils and butters is what helps this.

Sweet Almond Oil – Carrier Oil: Almond oil is a good source of vitamin E, which helps with dry hair, adds shine to dull hair, and strengthens weak hair. Effectiveness: When using almond oil, I usually just add a bit to my existing mixtures of oils/butters, so I don't want to say I know exactly what it does for my hair, or how much it would do all on its own. But I bought it because besides it being good for my hair, it has a pleasant fragrance and therefore makes everything I put in my hair smell good. Just being honest...

Tea Tree Oil – Essential Oil: Tea Tree Oil helps to unblock the sebaceous glands from buildup, as well as remove dead skin cells and other unwanted bacterial elements in your scalp, to promote the natural hair conditioning process and hair growth. It is also a very good treatment for dry, itchy scalp, and dandruff. Effectiveness: I initially started to use Tea Tree Oil because I read that it was really good at remedying an itchy scalp, and I suddenly found myself with that problem a while back. I knew nothing of its other great properties; I just went researching for this problem. I'd place a few drops of tea tree oil in a half bottle of shampoo to remedy the situation, and the few drops were all I needed; it's so concentrated, the entire bottle ends up smelling like Tea Tree Oil just from that very small amount. It worked for my itchy scalp very well. Then I noticed I got an added bonus: since I started using it, my scalp looked healthier. It's not greasy like what it used to look like when I tried to apply oils to it to combat dryness, but it's not dry anymore either. Just healthier, which is great. I now use it whether my scalp is itching or not, because it does great things for it.

Jojoba Oil – Carrier oil: One of the best oils for remedying hair loss, jojoba oil heals damaged hair by hydrating the hair from inside the cortex. It's antibacterial, and restores a good sebum balance in the hair by dissolving excess sebum and cleaning the scalp properly. It also calms the scalp. Effectiveness: Jojoba oil is a perfect addition to the combination of the oils I put in my hair and scalp. The thing I can see mostly is the hair seems to "drink" it in; although it is an oil, it does not leave my hair feeling greasy like other oils, and my hair looks and feels healthier when I add it to my hair. Something I don't stay without.

Rosemary Oil – Essential oil: Helps reduce and even reverse graying hair, and helps to stimulate and renew activity in hair bulbs. Effectiveness: Someone I knew that was natural before me told me about Rosemary's properties in reversing gray hair. I don't have many gray hairs, but the ones I do have are right in the very front of my hair on the hairline. I have been really bad lately at using the Rosemary, but I can definitely say that when I was using it regularly, I definitely saw a huge difference with my gray hair, to the point where I couldn't find them anymore. That's pretty impressive to me. The girl that told me about it told me the same thing was happening to her, and it reversed all her grays. It's important to note that I don't guarantee this for everyone, I'm just telling you MY story. Also we were both people who were JUST getting grays, which meant our hair probably still had some melanin in its strands. I don't know how well it will work for someone who's been gray for a long period of time. Also, I did not buy the rosemary oil (simply because I could not find it). I bought the actual rosemary leaves and put a TINY amount of water in it and boiled it. When I did, the oil drew right out of the leaves, and I mixed that warm, oily liquid in my conditioner and deep conditioned my hair. Since then, I found the rosemary oil and was putting that in my conditioner instead, but unfortunately, I have yet to see the changes I did with the natural leaves. So does it work? Based on research and my own experience, definitely; but for me, more so with the pure leaves than the bought oil.

Avocado Oil – Carrier oil: Avocado is ideal for dry hair. Avocado is full of healthy fats and vitamins your hair's needs. Effectiveness: Every once in a while, I give my hair an avocado deep condition. I buy the oil sometimes, but I prefer to simply mash the actual avocado into a paste and mix it in my conditioner mix, then apply it to my hair. It is GREAT for moisturizing – I can literally feel the difference in my hair for days after conditioning. Just make sure you fully wash it out of your hair during when rinsing. I use the avocado oil in my leave-in as well, and in my shea butter when I have some on hand.

Lavender Oil – Essential Oil: Known as an effective treatment for Hair loss (alopecia areata) and moisturizing and treating a dry scalp. Effectiveness: I have honestly only used lavender oil to make what I'm using in my hair smell good. It is such a calming aroma, since it has such great aromatherapy attributes, and is proven to improve sleep. But I've learned that it also calms the scalp itself; which is especially good when it has been traumatized by stress like heat, chemicals, etc.

Arnica Oil – Essential Oil: Stimulates the circulation in the scalp to help to promote hair growth and prevent premature hair loss. Effectiveness: I've never used this type of oil, so I can't attest to its effectiveness.

Bay Oil – Essential Oil: Good to restore dull looking hair. I've read that the best carrier oil to use would be jojoba oil, because they are a good mixture together. I have not, however, tried it myself.

Basil Oil – Essential oil: Stimulates scalp circulation, which promotes hair growth. Effectiveness: I've never used this type of oil.

Sage Oil – Essential oil: Darkens hair and helps with hair loss. Effectiveness: I personally have not used Sage, but know that many people mix Sage with Rosemary and claim it works wonders for their gray hairs. I'm inclined to believe them because of my experience with Rosemary, though I have yet to try the mixture.

Vegetable Glycerin: Glycerin is a humectant that is very good at drawing water from the air to moisturize your hair (or skin). It promotes moisture retention in hair, which can be helpful for those whose hair has the tendency to be dry or even coarse. Effectiveness: Glycerin is a two-sided coin. People can either really love glycerin, or really hate it. Ironically, both reasons are because it's that good at what it does. I personally believe your affinity of it will all depend on how you style you hair. If you are a natural-colored, curly haired person who is looking for something to moisturize your hair, glycerin gets rave reviews. It is VERY effective at moisturizing the hair because it draws water from the air and continually moisturizes the hair during the day. A little glycerin in your water mix can work wonders, as a little goes a long way (ranging from a few tbsps all the way to 1/8 of the bottle).

Now, for people who dye their hair or frequently use heat styling products (dryer, curling iron, flat iron, pressing comb, etc.), glycerin may not be loved as much. Glycerin conducts thermal energy VERY well (meaning it will transfer the heat from your curling/straightening device directly on to the hair) and that can cause heat damage. Also Glycerin is also known to strip color from your hair if it is dyed. This is because glycerin is a great solvent, so any dye in your hair that is not bound to the outside of your hair shaft will be easily captured by it, and absorbed. So, in closing, totally natural-haired people looking for constant moisture: most people recommend. Chemically, colored, or heat-altered hair: not so much. I personally only recently started using glycerin after my hair felt drier than usual when I started a consistent workout regimen. My sister raved about it, so I gave it a try. It was amazing. I saw immediate results. Usually when I wash my hair, I put leave-in products after conditioning and let my hair air dry, but the next day after it's fully dry, I would need to reapply. After adding glycerin to my products, I no longer need to do this – my hair remains moist, shiny and feels great to the touch the following day. It has also given me back the moisture in my hair that seemed to get lost after sweating so much from my daily workouts. So for me, it's a great product.

Carrot Oil: Strengthens and smoothes hair and adds shine. Rich in Vitamin A, E, and B-Carotene. Effectiveness: I used what I thought was carrot oil once (before I was natural), and I did not like the results, so it made me leery of it. The product I bought, however, turned out to not be a 100% natural product, so I don't know how much of what I didn't like was actually from the natural carrot oil, or the "additives" in the product itself. Carrot oil is known for being very greasy and heavy, but it is also known for being a great hot oil treatment (which is probably what I would use it for if I tried it again), and is really effective with repairing hair that is suffering from breakage and sealing split ends. Try it yourself, maybe being sparing with the portions initially.

This is just a breakdown of the products that I use or have heard good things about from others. It is by no means a complete list. Doing a little research can go a long way, but remember, don't fix something if it isn't broken. I haven't tried some of the oils that I've done research on; not because I don't think they are great products, but because hair likes consistency. It allows the hair to find its natural balance. Many times when you find a great product when your hair is relaxed, it works great at first, but after some time, it doesn't seem to work anymore. There are many reasons for this, but I won't get into them now. Natural hair doesn't work like this. Something has to change (like the weather or your location – which in turn changes the humidity and air your hair is used to) for your hair to suddenly not do well with the same regimen that had been working before. As a matter of fact, most naturals do adopt a different regimen for the summer months than in the winter. We will discuss that in a later section. But generally speaking, once you find a regimen that works for your hair, you can of course tweak it as you go and as NEEDED, but try to stay consistent, because consistency is best.

As far as different hair type needs, as I've mentioned many times in the past, natural hair has so many varieties and textures, it's difficult to generalize; but here is a small guide just to give you a starting point on where to begin:

For Hair in the Type 2 Category: The Type 2 wavy hair is usually light and finer in texture, and doesn't require any heavy products to weigh it down. Use mousses, light sprays and organic-based light gels to seal in moisture and define your hairstyle.

For Hair in the Type 3 Category: The type 3A and B curly hair is not too far from the Type 2 category, and doesn't fair well with heavy products. Use light crèmes and light gels to seal in moisture and define your curls. For 3B, because of your prone to frizziness, you may need something just a bit heavier, but not much, to offer a bit more control.

3C: 3C hair is, to me, right in the middle of everything. It doesn't have the same lightness, waviness, or sometimes even strength as the 3As or Bs, but it doesn't have as much shrinkage or kinks as the Type 4 category, or as much problem with dryness and breakage. Your hair however, has needs similar to the Type 4 Category, as it is a bit curlier, thirstier, and harder to manipulate than the earlier Type 3s. You should definitely incorporate products that have a creamy base instead of gels and mousses (except for Aloe Vera Gel, very good for the hair), along with creamy butters, light pomades, and oils for your 3C hair, depending on your individual needs.

Type 4 Category – This category needs heavier, thicker, creamier products to help seal in moisture and protect its strands. The hair should feel moist, but not wet or heavy (don't overdo it), and NEVER be in a state of dryness. If your hair feels like it needs a mist of water, you've waited too long to moisturize it. This is true for ALL categories, but because Type 4 hair is prone to breakage because the hair is very thirsty, people with this hair type need to be most careful with their retaining-moisture regimen. Remember, moisture comes only from water. You should use thick revitalizing crèmes, butters, pomades, and oils for the Type 4 Category.

*** Bonus – Leave-in recipe (for fine, dense hair, 4A–4B, to restore moisture) *:**

1/4 Cup Shea Butter

4 Tbsps of Olive Oil (Cold Pressed, Virgin)

1 Tbsp of Kinky Curly Knot Today

1 Tsp of Kuumba Cherry Mango Hair/Scalp Conditioner (or Oyin Handmade Burnt Sugar Pomade)

1 Tsp of Castor Oil

1 Tsp of Jojoba oil

1 Tsp of Coconut Oil

Mix together and apply to hair while it is still damp. Braid or style as desired.

*Measurements are just an approximation; use more or less as needed/desired.

Dying Your Natural Hair

Dying your hair can really give your natural hair a great look, but many (rightfully so) are leery of dyes and bleaches for their natural hair, because it can strip the hair and leave it dry and damaged. The safest things I know of to dye natural hair with are Henna dye or Indigo dye. There are some points, however, that you should be aware of:

Henna

Henna is an all-natural product and can actually be good for the hair, making it stronger and for some, softer. Some people have been known to use Henna strictly because of its benefits to the hair. Others have counteracted that repeated use of Henna could cause too much Henna to bind to the hair, closing your cuticles and weighing it down. I am not a hair coloring expert, so I would suggest that people do their own research to see if it's something you'd like to try.

FIRST THINGS FIRST. The only Henna that should be considered for use to dye your hair is Pure Henna. There are Henna compounds that people sell that can have damaging results on the hair. The only ingredient that should be in your Henna is "Lawsonia inermis," which is the actual original term for Henna. If it has anything else in the ingredients, then you have compound Henna, and using it can cause an adverse effect on your hair. The best Henna to use for your hair is body-art-quality Henna.

Henna only comes in ONE SHADE – that is an orange-red color. If you have a package that states a specific shade, like "Copper," "Auburn," or even "Black Henna," you do not have natural Henna and are taking a risk with your hair. Please do not let this fact lead you to believe, however, that everyone's hair will result in the same shade. What your original hair color is will strongly determine what shade your hair will actually turn out to be upon dying. You may want to do a strand test before you dye your entire head, to ensure you'll have results you'll want to live with, which goes to my next point...

Some people (like me, until I was educated) are under the impression that because Henna is an all-natural product, it will fade with time. This is totally untrue. Henna is a permanent dye, and has to grow out and the dyed hair cut off, if you want to be rid of it. Please keep that in mind before dying.

Indigo

Indigo is also a natural product, and is the same dye used for dying really dark blue jeans (Indigo jeans). If your hair is already dark, it can be used to achieve that very dark, "blue-black" color. Some suggest doing a Henna treatment first to give the Indigo dye something to attach itself to for a better result; people who use it have also said that using the Henna first gives the hair a better chance of turning out black, rather than with a bluish hue. Others mix smaller, varying amounts of Indigo with the Henna to achieve different, darker shades for the Henna coloring in your hair.

Again, this is just basic information; please do your own research and/or consult a hair professional when using these products.

*** Other decent color options to research:**

– *EcoColors Hair Color*

– *Tints of Nature*

– *Palette By Nature*

Caring For Your Natural Hair: All Alcohols are Not Created Equal

Most people know that alcohol is not good for your hair. It sucks out all the moisture from your hair, and makes it dry and brittle. There are, however, some "alcohols" that don't create this result. As a matter of fact, they do the exact opposite.

I bought this product a while back that I really liked: Organic Root Stimulator Olive Oil Smooth Pudding. It's a great product for giving you a hold that is not stiff at all, just enough to keep your edges smooth if you have it in a ponytail, bun, or something similar. It doesn't flake like gel, doesn't leave a residue, and also smells great. At any rate, I found this product shortly before a time when I was becoming more conscious of what products I put in my hair. So one day, I decided to read what was in it, and I saw "Cetearyl Alcohol." I was crushed! I loved this product and it has alcohol? But I just couldn't understand it. The product didn't dry out my hair at all, how could it have alcohol? So I decided to do a little research on that particular type of alcohol, and found out some interesting facts:

Alcohol isn't just one substance, but actually different categories of alcohols: a) Alcohols that are drying to the skin and hair: Ethanol, SD alcohol, Alcohol Denat, Propanol, Propyl Alcohol and Isopropyl (rubbing) Alcohol; b) Alcohol that is put in spirits to consume orally; c) Miscellaneous alcohols: Benzyl alcohol is generally neither good nor bad for your hair, just merely used as a preservative in products, and Propylene glycol is used as a humectant, (something that draws water from the air and moisturizes the hair); and finally, d) Fatty alcohols that are derived from natural sources like oils, fats, plants, and animals. These types of alcohols are actually good for the hair and skin. It's the last type of alcohol that we will discuss here. There are quite a few of these fatty alcohols that are in this category: Lauryl Alcohol, Myristyl Alcohol, Behenyl Alcohol, Cetearyl Alcohol, Cetyl Alcohol, and Stearyl Alcohol. I will break down the last two:

Cetyl alcohol: This is a fatty alcohol that used to be derived from whale oil, but is now principally derived from vegetable oils like coconut and palm oils. This alcohol is used as an emollient (making the skin and hair softer), an emulsifier (making oils and water bind together), and a surfactant (making a product easier to spread and apply). This is a good ingredient to find in your hair products.

Stearyl alcohol: This fatty alcohol is a waxy solid alcohol obtained from whale or dolphin oil and used as a lubricant, and meant to slow down the evaporation of water.

There are also mixtures of the above fatty alcohols that are also good for the hair. Examples are: Cetearyl Alcohol, Cetostearyl Alcohol, Lauryl-Myristyl Alcohol, and Cetyl-Stearyl Alcohol, among others. So, in closing, before you throw away a product because you see the word "alcohol," please remember, all alcohols are not created equal.

Caring For Your Natural Hair: PH Balance and Restoring Porous Hair

Although most of us don't think about it much, the PH balance in our hair is very important for our hair's health. Our hair naturally produces sebum that helps to maintain the proper PH. The PH balance in our hair, however, can be affected by a change in the weather, and (most importantly) the products we put in our hair. The PH scale encompasses two extremes: Alkaline and Acidity. The scale is from 0 (strongly Acidic) to 14 (Strongly Alkaline). Having a level of 7 represents neutrality (water is at a 7). A natural PH balance in healthy hair falls between a 4.5 and a 5.5.

Some products mention on their bottles what their PH level is, some do not. If you are using store-bought products that have a high PH level (more alkaline), the cuticles in the hair follicles become open (instead of lying down and protecting the hair, while sealing the moisture in). This causes the hair to soak up everything you apply to it, while at the same time, lose the ability retain the moisture it takes in. This type of condition is described as porous hair. The high PH products also strip the hair of its natural oils. The result of all of this is dry, brittle, weak hair that looks dull (because the cuticles aren't lying down and reflecting light), and hair that breaks easily. You would then have to correct it with something that contains a lower PH (more acidic) to balance it out. Because some products don't give you their PH information, some people go as far as to buy litmus paper to test the PH balance of the products they use.

I'm going to be totally honest here. I am really not a fan of trying something just because it works great for someone else, and I try not to fix what isn't broken with my own hair. Because I don't use many store-bought products and I nourish my hair with natural oils, butters, and plant derivatives, I don't worry too much about my PH balance. Also, Aloe Vera is known for balancing and maintaining your

PH, and it is the first thing I put in my leave-in conditioner mix right after I shampoo and condition my hair. I can literally see the difference in my hair when I apply it. Finally, because of the protective styles I wear (to protect it from the air) and the lack of too many other factors to alter my hair (like heat, styling gels, store-bought products, etc.), I don't have PH problems. But everyone doesn't have the same hair condition, nor do they all use the same regimen, so knowing how to restore your PH is very important information to have.

Because apple cider vinegar is slightly acidic, many use it as an acidic rinse to restore their hair's natural PH balance after shampooing. To do this, dilute the vinegar with water (distilled water if possible) – 1 part Vinegar to 5 parts water, and pour the mixture on your head. Leave it in for about 15 minutes, then lightly rinse it out. The apple cider vinegar also closes the cuticles as it removes residue from the hair, so many women use it often. Others only use it as needed, or when their hair is in a porous state. With so many types of curly hair, you need to personally determine what's right for you.

Caring For Your Natural Hair: Your Ends and Protective Styles

I've already discussed hair growth. Your hair already grows. Retaining the ends of your hair is what gives your hair "growth" that is visual. Your hair can grow and grow, *and* grow (like it is now), but if you don't actually retain the growth, the length of your hair will remain the same. Let's talk about how to retain that growth. The ends of your hair are the oldest part of your hair, and require special attention. It is the part of your hair that gets the least amount of sebum, the part of your hair that rubs and suffers from friction on your clothes, and the part that is susceptible to drying, splitting, breaking, snapping off, etc. In addition, your hair is prone to breakage from many different elements like the sun, changes in the weather, the products you use, even the air and wind. It is most advantageous for you to be aware of its vulnerability, and take care of it accordingly:

- When applying conditioner, product, styling etc., your ends should always be in your mind. Pay special attention to them when applying product to your hair to ensure they are fully nourished, and when doing different hairstyles, keep in mind that protected ends (tucked in, braided, twisted, or pinned up and inside) are far more likely to be retained.

- When your hair reaches shoulder length, it is very vulnerable to breakage, and will be until it reaches a little ways past your shoulders. The air tends to dry out your ends before the rest of your hair, and much like why you wouldn't wear a cotton scarf on your head at night, when you leave your hair out to brush on your shoulders, the friction from rubbing against your clothes (biggest problem) causes split ends and it breaks off. It also gets caught on things like necklaces on the back of your neck. During this vulnerable time, try to wear your hair in protective styles as often as possible (as a general rule, you should wear your hair in protective styles more often than not at any length, but it is especially important at this time). Some suggestions are:

91

- Buns
- Single Braids
- Cornrows
- Single Twists
- Flat Twists
- Bantu knots
- Pinned up
- Extensions
- Wigs
- Weaves (with your hair BRAIDED underneath; no bonds or glues)

Please be careful not to do the following:

- Don't wear tight ponytails, braids, or buns. Basically anything that is pulling your hair too much. Even when locking hair, you shouldn't pull it too tight, or the tension can slowly pull out the hair to the point where the lock can actually pop off, or even pull out from the root of your hair.

- Don't use rubber bands in your hair – use coated bands. This one we should already know.

- Don't pull hair clips out of the hair and use hair accessories that can pinch, snag, or pull the hair. Be careful to slowly remove ANY accessory from the hair.

- Don't use coated bands or headbands that have a metal clasp in them (the hair gets caught and pulls out in the clasps while you're removing them from the hair).

- Don't use Metal Clips. Besides your hair getting caught in them, because of the moisture-filled products you would now use in your natural hair, the metal tends to rust. A good option for this and conventional hairpins are 'good day hairpins,' a less-harsh option for the hair.

- Try not to get your hair caught in the knot of your head scarf. Something as simple as this is a common reason for hair loss/breakage in the back of your head. After tying the scarf, be sure to run your finger in between the scarf and hair to confirm no hair has been inadvertently caught in the knot of the scarf, which can pull and snap off while you move in your sleep.

Besides protecting your hair, protective styles actually are very effective in helping your hair retain moisture. This is easily identified when comparing hair that has been braided in big braids: if you examine the part of the hair that was in a braid, versus the part of the hair from the scalp all the way *to* the braid, there is a clear difference in how it feels and how much moisture was retained.

Many people ask me, what is the sense of growing your hair so long and beautiful if you can't show it off? If your hair is always tucked in and hidden away, how can you enjoy it? Honestly, I think choices like these are things that we deal with when it comes to our hair, regardless. For example, many women love the flat iron and the curling iron, but we know that if we use it every day, we will pay the price that comes with it. Same for dyes, rinses, texturizers, glue-ins and everything else. Can you wear your hair out? Of course you can. You just need to know that the more you wear it out, the more chances you can have of breakage and damage. Plain and simple. Everyone maintains their own balance, and what's comfortable for them. I flat-iron my hair maybe three to four times a year. Some do it once a month. Some do it once a year. There's nothing set in stone, it's whatever is comfortable for you, and how much you think your hair can deal with. Do I think my hair can deal with more than four times a year? Sure. But I'm not comfortable with it, so I don't do it any more than that. And when I DO flat-iron it, I prepare my hair for it by doing many steps over the course of a few days. I have a forum every month, and I wear my hair out and curly for almost every forum (I do twist outs, I love them), and also when I go out. That's totally fine for me. Weekends are also when I take my twists out and enjoy my hair before I wash it. But will I go to work on a daily basis with my hair out? Never. Have I done it once in a while? Yes! No one is telling you not to enjoy your hair. Just be very aware that there are consequences to how you treat your hair on a daily basis. It's all about moderation.

Caring For Your Natural Hair: Heat Styling and Resisting the Urge

As we go natural and our hair becomes strong and grows out to beautiful lengths, some of us see how long and beautiful our hair is when it's straight, and get the urge to revert back to our old ways of either relaxing it or straightening it, and leaving it out all the time. We reason that since our hair is now healthy, we can relax our hair in this state and just work on maintaining that healthy condition. Or if we don't relax it, we can straighten it with heat on a regular basis, and we're still natural, so the hair will be fine.

Everyone is entitled to choice, and it's your hair. But you now know what it is you're actually doing to your hair when you relax it. Is it worth it?

Well let's say you're past that point. Your mind is made up, and you go out and get a relaxer and get the exact results you are looking for: Straight, long hair. That's fine. Just know that from the very moment you relax your hair, on the inside, it is damaged. Over time, the hair gets thinner and thinner, and weaker and weaker. It breaks, it sheds, and it's lacking moisture. This is why when the new growth grows out, the natural hair is literally starving for moisture in the harsh environment that the relaxer has created; resulting in coarse, dry, brittle, hard to manage hair. I personally know two friends who were natural, their hair grew long and beautiful. They then relaxed it, and within a year, they had to cut it off because their hair broke off due to damage. And each one said beforehand, "That's not going to happen to me. I'm just going to take care of it really well, so it doesn't get damaged." Not realizing that the hair was damaged from the time they left the beautician. So please think long and hard before you make a decision that can make you have to start from scratch.

For people that use heat-styling methods to straighten their natural hair on a regular basis, know that although you are using a temporary solution to straighten your hair, and this can be ok if used sparingly, the fact is that heat styling is one of the leading causes of damaged hair (in any kind of hair). Heat damages the hair's cuticles and pulls out the inner moisture from it. The results can be dry, damaged, brittle hair. ALSO in natural hair, there are many, many cases that I'm aware of where too much heat permanently breaks down the cross-bonds, and when you try to revert your hair back to the curls, it does NOT revert back. Some have been successful at getting it to come back after several protein treatments and deep conditioning, but others have not been so lucky. Overall, make it an indulgence to straighten your hair to sport the full length of your hair, or to use any kind of heat for a new hairstyle every once in a while. Do it with the knowledge you now have about what can happen to your hair. Be sure to behave knowingly, don't overdo it, and act accordingly (take precautions).

When you do use heat, PLEASE prepare your hair for it with a deep conditioner or a protein treatment, and PLEASE USE A HEAT PROTECTANT. Me, personally, when I straighten my hair, the process runs over the course of days. The first day, I give my hair a wash and a serious deep conditioning. When done, I add my leave-in treatment and my heat protectant (the heat protectant has to have time to bond to your hair in order to protect it, other-wise it just burns off with the heat). I don't use heat the same day because it's already been washed and conditioned, and it's just too much for one day. So I braid it in big sections to start stretching out the hair, then let it air dry as usual. The next day, I use a blow dry-er on warm or low (not hot) heat to help stretch out the curls even further. This way, the flat iron is not left with a lot of work to do.

I use a ceramic or tourmaline flat iron – reason being it distributes the heat on the iron better, so you don't end up with 'hot spots' that burn your hair. If you can smell your hair while you're flat-ironing it, it is burning. I used to think that smell was perfectly normal. Now I would cringe if I smelled it. I part my hair in very small sections so that I can straighten the hair without having to continually reapply the flat iron on one spot, or repeatedly go over the same section (something else I regarded as normal). You also need to hold the ends of the hair taut (stretched) to add tension the further you get down to the ends; otherwise, you'll end up with frizzy ends that don't straighten. Some use a clamp to hold the ends of the hair, which, in my opinion, is best.

I then wrap it overnight or for most of the day; or, something I've started doing recently, I wear it in a bun similar to a bantu knot – it's twisted all the way around to the end and held with a soft scrunchie. When I take it out, the hair is completely straight, but has big waves in it, which I like. This way, whatever isn't lying down completely straight when I'm done flat-ironing, by the time I take it out of my wrap or bun, my hair is completely straight, flowing and very shiny. It takes a long time, but it's well worth it for me to keep my hair healthy during the process. Using bantu knots also prevents me from having to use more heat for curls or waves:

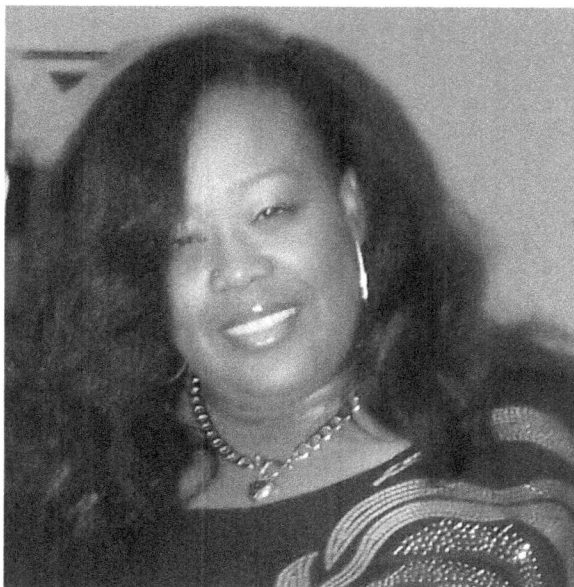

This look was done with app. 4-6 bantu knots after straightening, left in for a few hrs.

Natural Women Wearing Wigs and Weaves

The question was posed to me some time ago, "How do you feel about people who are natural, yet wear wigs and weaves?" Do I think they're being fake, phony, or being hypocrites? The simple answer, in my opinion of course, is no; but this question is rooted once again behind your reasoning for wearing wigs and weaves in the first place. Wigs and weaves can be used as protective styles. Some swear by them in the wintertime when the weather can be most harsh on their hair. Some turn to them when they are first transitioning, and usually wear cornrows underneath. Some wear them to give their hair a break from extension braids. Some even wear them because they feel like wearing a straight hairstyle one day, but don't want to put their hair through the heat process. I honestly don't see anything wrong with any of these. You know who you are and anyone who knows you knows who you are as well. This is just a protective style choice, or simply a style change. It doesn't make you phony, nor does it make you send the wrong message. The world we live in is one filled with options. The idea of exercising them is totally fine.

Now, when you're wearing your hair in a weave or a wig because you don't think your own hair is an option, besides a BC, that to me is different. I heard someone say recently that if you're natural but you either press your hair straight every day or wear a wig or a weave all the time, to the point where no one even KNOWS you're natural, then you're not really natural. I will have to say that I agree with that statement. If you've made the decision to go "natural," but you never actually wear your hair natural, then you're not really representing yourself as a natural-haired person. It's kind of like a person that has turned Rasta (Rastafarian), but no one knows they're a Rasta, because they don't like the way it looks, or they feel that in order to go outside, they have to wear a wig because it's not visually acceptable. Can you really call yourself a Rasta if you're intentionally hiding it? This can be a very controversial subject; people can get very defensive about it and sometimes, the answer to the conflict comes down to an individual's simple choice. If you think about it, almost everyone does things to enhance their natural appearance, right? We pluck our eyebrows, we wear makeup, we wax our body hair, etc.; and all of these things are altering our natural selves to some degree, so people shouldn't be so judgmental. Men and women alike do things to groom and enhance their looks. But like everything else in this world, there should be a balance in all we do. If someone wore makeup or shaped their eyebrows and still looked like themselves – just a bit more "refined" – it would be perfectly acceptable and simply perceived as one enhancing what is already there. If someone caked on an obscene amount of make-up every day, however, it would not be viewed in the same manner. The difference is distinctive: there's enhancement, and then there's someone in hiding.

Whatever you do in this world, you should be able to stand by it and be proud of your choices. What's the sense of doing it if you can't? For people who go natural and wear wigs all the time, press their hair, or wear weaves all the time, I would say (and this is only my opinion) that these are people who recognize that relaxers are very damaging to their hair or may have even experienced hair damage from a relaxer and have decided to make a change. They still haven't, however, fully embraced being natural, or still may not even like the idea of being natural. I was there myself. Well first and foremost, to those people, I say be YOU. Don't go out there and sport an afro to prove a point to anyone. I will say though that if you don't eventually embrace your natural hair, you'll be missing out on the best part of being natural, because you'll never actually reach your hair's full potential. You'll never discover how beautiful your hair is or can be, how versatile it is, how stylish you can wear it or how long it can grow. For some people, that's totally fine with them. To which I say, then that's fine with me.

Now for those opposed to the wigs, weaves and the like overall, I do understand where some are coming from in the sense that we are supposed to be encouraging to our fellow curly-haired sisters, embrace our hair, showcase it, and be proud of it! And I'm with you on that! I just don't think that wearing a wig, weave or even a press on occasion takes away from that. Who we are is going to shine through, regardless! I normally wear my hair in twists or braids to work, occasionally wearing it out curly once in a blue moon. But three or four times a year, I flat-iron my hair. If I was to wear my straightened hair to work on one of these days, do you think that people would think I was being untrue to my natural self? Not at all. Anyone that knows me knows I'll be right back to my usual curly-haired self in a couple of days. There's also the fact that embracing your hair does not happen in a day. Going natural, for some, is a major, major change to your overall look. Besides having to either cut all your hair off or transition, you have to essentially learn how to care for your hair all over again. This requires a great deal of trial and error, patience and experimenting. Many will not get it right immediately. So for some (including myself at the time), you are really just trying your best to get through this difficult phase. Doesn't exactly exude someone who is embracing their new look, right? So you may want to, until you figure it all out, wear a weave or a wig to protect the hair until you're comfortable that you know how to care for it, or even style it. Do I think I need to flat-iron my hair for every special occasion? Absolutely not, because I love my hair; it's thick, it's curly, it's defined, it's natural and it's beautiful. Did I think that way in the very beginning? ABSOLUTELY NOT! I didn't know what I was doing, and my hair was a MESS. I only didn't opt to wear wigs or weaves because I've never cared for them, even when I had a relaxer. Weaves I've tried, and always ended up wanting to take them out in a few short days, which would end up being a waste of money. Wigs feel like a helmet on my head and make me want to itch. Honestly, I didn't care for the braids too much either, but I had been able to wear braids in the past, and it was the closest thing to me that I felt I could do and be myself. So for me, it was the best choice. Lastly, there are a lot of options for wigs and weaves now. You can get a wig that is closer to your own hair texture. I know a girl who is natural, but she loves to experiment with color. She's just not willing to put her hair through that. So she gets partial synthetic wigs (where the front of your hair is showing and blends in with the wig) that are very close to her own curl pattern. This is her way of enjoying a color change without hurting her natural curls. She interchanges them all the time and has fun. And everyone still knows that she is natural, because she also wears her own hair as well, and they look very similar.

If you do opt to wear a wig, know that wigs can be damaging to the hair, especially near the hairline. Please incorporate certain precautions when using:

Look for wigs that are made on a net base that allow your scalp to breathe. For the conventional wig, try not to put the comb directly on the hairline and look for wigs that have a drawstring. Wear it a few inches from the hairline, or use bobby pins to help secure it and put the comb on the wig cap, not the hair. Your hair should not be loose under a wig, and left vulnerable to friction. Please braid the hair so that it can stay protected and retain moisture better.

The conventional nylon wig cap or one made of cotton is really not good for your hair, and shouldn't be used when growing out your hair, for the same reasons you wouldn't wear it as a scarf at night. Many use a men's satin cap, wave cap or a doo-rag. If you use this method, be sure to secure your wigs with pins. Others use no cap at all if their hair is in braids and protected. I have read about the comfy grip, a gel-filled headband that distributes the heat under the wig better while keeping the wig in place, but I have not personally heard of anyone trying it or their results.

For lace wigs that you are gluing on, do not glue the wigs directly on the hairline; glue is damaging to the hair and can pull out the delicate hair along the hairline. I honestly would not recommend you gluing anything on at all, unless it's a weave onto a wig cap that can come off. The scalp needs to be able to breathe, so it can get proper circulation, and gluing it on suggests you won't be taking it off for long periods at a time.

You also need to be able to get to the hair to moisturize it. Moisturize very, very often. Hair underneath a wig can get very dry. Pay extra attention to the hair at the hairline as well. Some wash more often, others will even moisturize, then put on a baggy underneath. This however, you should practice with caution; a wet scalp underneath a hot wig can cause adverse effects, like a rash, bacteria, hair loss and otherwise. The key is to remember that the scalp needs to breath, no matter what regimen you decide on.

Caring For Your Natural Hair: The "Hands Disease"

The "hands disease" or "hands-in-hair disease" is not a real disease, rather it's a term coined in the natural-haired community for people who can't keep their hands out of their hair. It is one of the subtlest things we unconsciously do that breaks off our hair. Constant pulling, twisting, curling between our fingers, and tugging of the hair make our strands fragile, and slowly break off the hair. Sometimes, even without changing anything else, just learning to leave your hair alone for an extended period of time works wonders for your hair retention.

I, admittedly, have this disease (smile). When I first went natural, it was very new, a little strange, and I was also a bit nervous of how people received my new look. Because of this, I was always looking at or "fixing" my hair (not really, just touching and pulling on the curls). This however, was only an issue when I left my hair out. When I braided, twisted or pinned up my hair and it was tucked away and protected, I didn't have the same desire to play in it. So wearing my hair in protective styles, for me, is not only to protect my hair from external elements, but also from myself!

When your hair is out, please be conscious of having your hands in your hair all of the time. If you can't control this habit yet, try to keep your hair in styles that make it hard for you to get to your hair. If you're like me, the protective styles take away the desire to play in it anyway. And once your hair reaches a certain length and you're used your natural curls, for some, this desire goes away with time.

Caring For Your Natural Hair: Hairdressers

Admittedly, I am what you might call a "do-it-yourself" natural-haired person. Until recently, I had never even gone to a hairdresser since I've been natural. No one, in my opinion, can care for your hair better than you, once you learn how. With your own hands, you know exactly what's going in your hair, you have the patience to comb your hair in a non-abusive way because it's *your* hair and you care about the health of it, and you should not be using heat in your hair on a frequent basis for any reason. Also, if your hair is thick or tightly coiled, you should not be using a small, fine-toothed comb that can pull out the hair you've taken so much time to grow. Another factor to consider is natural hair products and oils are not cheap. You might want to spend your money on quality products for your hair every month, than on hairdressers to simply wash and style your hair every week..

Now with that said, I do understand and appreciate the knowledge and advice of a professional. If you have a special occasion and want a professional to give you a great style, or if you are the type of woman that would rather have a salon take care of your hair, there are great, knowledgeable (key word here), natural hair care salons that can take care of your hair, and even help to educate you on caring for your curls or locks. Regular hairdressers you went to when you were relaxed for wash and sets, perms, etc., are simply not great options anymore. The idea of going to a standard, everyday hairdresser, now that I am natural, is not an option for me, period. Your natural hair needs time, patience, and *more* time and patience to be cared for. A regular hairdresser (ahem, sorry. *Most* regular hairdressers) don't have that kind of time. The average hairdresser is not going to have the patience to sit there and divide your hair into sections, slowly detangle knots, or wash your hair the way it should be washed or even dried. They have a business to run and other clients waiting, so they have to find that balance of making you feel special, while still catering to everyone else. This usually entails making you look good, and moving on. Notice how I said, making you "look good." What makes you "look good," however, is not always what's healthy for your natural hair, or any type of hair for that matter. They're going to want to use heat often to achieve a certain style. They're likely to use a fine, rat-tail comb to comb out your tresses. Even if you bring in your own shampoo and conditioner, they're going to want to use commercial products like gel and setting lotion in your hair that are, once again, made to make you "look good" and may not be healthy for your hair.

Natural hairstylists, on the other hand, have experience in dealing with different hair types, removing frizz, defining and stretching your curls, shaping the hair, etc. My recent visit to Natural Trendsetters in Florida left me with a bit more knowledge on how to stretch and curl my hair, and they didn't even use heat during my visit, except when putting me under a dryer with a cap for deep conditioning. I was able to wear the rod style for a week, even after I combed it out and was braiding it at night. It was well worth the trip, and I didn't feel like my hair was being abused.

Unfortunately, they're not always as easy to find as a regular hairdresser, but we live in a digital world, so take some time, look around, and seek them out. Don't go to a hairdresser that tells you "we also deal with natural hair." Go to an expert, if you can find one. But please be careful and do your research. Just because some hairdressers say they cater to natural hair doesn't guarantee they won't practice the same methods as regular salons; do your research and make sure you find other natural-haired clients that can tell you about their personal experiences, or search the web (not the company site) for unbiased client reviews.

Caring For Your Natural Hair: Sleep Regimen

The good thing about a proper sleep regimen for our hair is, for most people of color, we already know one thing: we should always go to bed with our hair protected in a satin scarf, wrap or bonnet, or even use a satin pillowcase. The simple reasons being that resting our heads on absorbable cotton or other materials causes the natural oils to be absorbed from our hair into our bedding, and as we naturally toss and turn at night, the constant friction from rubbing our hair on the pillowcase material causes our hair to tangle and break, and we end up losing our precious ends.

For people going natural, I will add one more factor. Our hair does much better if we keep our hair braided, twisted, Bantu-knotted, or some other sort of protective style that keeps the hair from being out and loose. Besides protecting your ends, it keeps the hair moisturized, detangled, and easier to manage. Even when I am wearing twist outs going into the next day, I will, very loosely, flat twist my hair in big sections when going to bed. The twist outs not only keep their shape, they actually stretch out a bit and look even better the next day. I still had on a scarf, but went to bed ONE time without braiding or twisting my hair up. It was the first time, and the last. My hair was so dry, compacted, tangled and knotted up the next morning that I had to spend a great deal of time detangling it and reapplying products to it. For the health of your hair, please apply this habit to your nightly regimen. If you really don't want to braid or twist the hair (or something similar), at least place the hair in a loose bun. Even if there's a chance your hair won't stay as moisturized as the other options, it won't be tangled, frizzy, or have a chance to get compacted and abused throughout the night.

Caring For Your Natural Hair: Applying Extensions

Extensions are a great option to use when you're transitioning or have recently done your big chop. If done properly, the small amount of tension promotes hair growth, the braids keeps the hair protected from exterior elements, and it is a great way to give your hair a break from combing and brushing. I used braids a great deal when I first did my Big Chop, and I do not regret this, because I saw a great deal of growth while keeping my hair in braids. There are a few things that you should definitely know when applying extensions:

- You should use synthetic kanekalon hair. It is a higher quality of synthetic hair, it keeps curls or waves if the style is applied with hot water, and it has a better absorption rate than other synthetics or even other types of human hair; as most of you know, we generally don't buy human hair of our own texture, many buy human hair from other races to apply to their hair.

- If your scalp is sensitive, you may want to pre-treat the synthetic hair with an acidic vinegar rinse. Just take the hair and place it in a sink or bowl filled with warm water and 1 cup of distilled vinegar for 15-20 minutes. You should be able to see a thin film appear on the surface of the water. If so, you've achieved the desired results. Remove the hair from the bowl and hang it somewhere to dry, then use it to braid as usual. It may leave a slight smell in the hair, but like when doing acidic rinses in your own hair, this should pass within a short amount of time.

- When braiding your hair in box (or single) braids or twists, you don't want to braid your hair too small. This is a very common mistake that results in hair loss and breakage. You are adding weight to your strands by adding more hair. You don't want to braid your hair in sections that are too small to carry this weight, or that would put too much extra strain on the scalp. This is a crucial tip to hair retention, especially near the delicate hairline. The individual sections should each be a thick enough lock of hair so the hair can stay strong and healthy in the braids. The thinner or finer your hair, the bigger the sections for the braids should be as well.

- Do not add too much synthetic hair to each braid. Same concept applies as above. It adds too much stress to your scalp for too much weight to be added to each strand of your own hair. A good indicator is how well the braid is able to transition from where your hair ends to where there is only synthetic hair in the braid. If it goes from very fat to skinny, there is too much hair in one braid. It should look like a normal braid, generally close to even along the entire strand.

- Another suggestion is to braid the hair by using your lock of hair as one of the three strands you're braiding. It keeps your hair in the braid as one strong lock of hair, and is more effective in hair retention. When you reach the end of your hair, simply split one of the other synthetic strands and continue braiding. The less strain on your scalp, the better it is for hair retention and growth.

- Do not braid the hair too tight. This causes unneeded stress to the hair and the scalp, and can result in hair loss. You shouldn't do anything in your hair so tight that it causes excessive tension – braids, ponytails or otherwise.

- You need to lightly mist and fortify your hair with water and a good braid spray or oils of your choice on a constant basis. You should NOT leave your hair to become too dry while in braids. Mist the hair all the way to where your hair ends. Your hair should always be moisturized while in this condition. I did not mist my hair every day, but every other day. Practice whatever works for you to keep your hair in a constant moisturized condition, based on your hair type.

Many people do not wash their hair while it is in braids. Some say the braids will get too frizzy and not look good anymore. But you will not be washing and conditioning your hair the way you did in the past, so this should not be a problem (please see Shampooing and Conditioning section). You can use a natural sea sponge (or similar) or a soft cloth (like a baby's rag) to wash your hair while it is in braids, so that your scalp stays clean and is in a healthy state to grow. As usual, do not scratch the hair or scalp, or rub a towel through it when drying. For me, washing my braids this way actually revitalized my braids and made them look shiny and newer again because the hair was clean.

Sometimes when you remove the extensions, you will find a white, dusty film wrapped around the root of your hair. It is usually isolated to the braids near the hairline. This is product that has settled at the hairline and dried in your hair, locked in with dust and dirt from the air. The problem becomes bigger the longer the braids are in your hair. This is perfectly normal, even when you wash the hair; but it is also the reason most will suggest that you don't keep braids in longer than 8 weeks, because if this film becomes too locked or tangled in the hair, it becomes difficult to remove and can cause breakage. Some people make it a point not to apply too much oil, or spray too much along the hairline, to avoid or reduce this. When it happens, please do not rip your hair out trying to remove this from your hair. Slowly work this out of your hair. Some people wet the hair, or use conditioner or another product that has a great deal of slippage, so it is easier to slide this film out of the hair. Whatever you do, please take your time. My technique is to take only a few strands of hair out of the film at a time, until most of it is out. I do this slowly so I don't break the hair. It then becomes easier to slide the rest out of the remainder of hair.

If done well and properly cared for, hair that is left in extensions can increase hair growth and leave the hair in a thicker, longer, and healthier state.

Caring For Your Natural Hair: Combating Knots

Many in the natural hair community, at one point and time, have suffered from knots. Whether they be single-strand knots (some call them fairy knots), or two or more strands that have knotted together, it is something that comes up often, and I get a great deal of questions about them.

There are many things that contribute to knots in the hair, but many of the knots generally happen because of the simple fact that our hair is so curly, curls constantly meet with other curls, fold over each other and form a knot, or knot around its own strand. This is something not easily solved, but can at least be controlled in a few ways:

- Friction causes knots. Sleeping with a satin scarf or on a satin pillow and wearing protective styles combats this.

- Don't leave clips and barrettes in your hair at night; they can get tangled in the hair and cause knots when you take them out.

- Split ends also cause knots, and should be trimmed regularly; not only for this reason, but to keep your hair in a healthy state.

- Knots occur often while washing your hair the conventional way. Try not to wash your hair by piling it on top of your head and rubbing vigorously. Instead, braid your hair loosely in sections and wash it gently with a sea sponge or soft baby cloth.

- If you leave your hair loose after washing, it will shrink up to its full curl capacity. When the hair is stretched after washing (pulled straighter than your regular curl would shrink), whether with braiding, curling, twisting, or otherwise, it has a less frequency to knot up because the stretched out curls and have less opportunity to tangle up with each other, or in its own strand.

- Knots are able to be detangled better when you comb your hair from the ends and work your way up.

- The more your hair is left out loose, the more your hair will tangle. Wear your hair in protective styles (at night as well), and you will have a lot less knots to speak of. Because I generally wear my hair in protective styles, I don't have a big problem with knots anymore.

- When the hair is dry, it tangles easier. Please keep the hair moisturized. Deep condition often, and please do not comb the hair while it is completely dry; mist it lightly with your water solution before combing.

When you do get knots, slippage and patience is the key to detangling them without taking out your hair. Detangle in the shower with conditioner in your hair so the knots slide out of each other, rather than getting more tangled. If you're not in the shower, apply a little leave-in conditioner, oil, or a creamy hair product to the knot before trying to take it out, and exercise a bit of patience. You can also try these points:

- You can use a pin to slowly work the hair out of a tight knot. This requires patience, and possibly a mirror if you can't see the hair in your hand.

- If you have really stubborn knots that won't move, you can try applying conditioner or oil and leaving it in overnight, giving the hair a chance to really moisturize and loosen the knots.

- When all else fails, slowly remove all of the hair that can be removed from the knot (usually only one or two strands remain), and take a scissors and clip the knot off. DON'T just pull it out and break your hair, possibly from the root. Save as much of the healthy hair as possible. Sometimes you can even work the knot further to the end of the hair, even if you can't get it out. Then cut it off. But oftentimes if it can move, it can be detangled.

Caring For Your Natural Hair: Daily Diet

Your hair needs certain vitamins and minerals for it to be healthy, and although you can add natural oils and products externally, the vitamins also should come from within your diet. The following are foods that are rich in vitamins and/or minerals that promote healthy hair. If you're not going to eat these things, it would be advisable to take a daily multivitamin to supplement your diet.

Key things to add to your diet to promote hair growth:

Eggs, Lean Meats (beef poultry, liver), green leafy vegetables, broccoli, yellow vegetables, nuts, avocado, dairy products, and a lot of water.

Essential fatty acids (flaxseed oil, evening primrose oil, deep/cold water fish, cod liver oil, and salmon oil) improve the actual texture of the hair. They prevent the hair from being dry and brittle.

The following are key vitamins used to promote hair growth, strengthen hair strands, thicken hair, and prolong the hair's natural color:

Vitamin A – needed to produce sebum.

Vitamin B and B-Complex Vitamins – Vitamin B vitamins are the most effective vitamins to promote hair growth and health: Niacin–B-3, Panthenol–B-5, B-6, B-12, and Biotin–B-7 (thickens the hair).

Vitamin E – necessary for good blood circulation in the scalp, beneficial in preventing hair loss.

Copper – produces melanin and prolongs your original hair color.

Vitamin C and Zinc – required for the body to develop collagen, which is needed for strong hair.

Incorporating these things in your diet not only aids in healthy hair and hair growth, but is also good for your skin, nails, and overall health, for a great body and active lifestyle.

Caring For Your Natural Hair: Combating Weather Changes

Extreme weather can damage your hair. Whether it's extreme heat or extreme cold, weather changes can affect our hair, and we need to change up our routine to protect our strands during these times.

In the winter months, we have to deal with the air outside that is very cold and harsh, and at the same time, bear the heat in our house that isn't natural heat. Both things are very drying to the hair, so we need to combat this:

Start internally: Essential fatty acids found in Omega 3s, olive oil (extra virgin), flax oil, fish, etc., provide natural waterproofing that seals in moisture in the hair. Also, we need to fortify the hair a little more than normal: More deep conditioning, Hot oil treatments, and use thicker butters (like shea) or more oils. Avoid blow-drying or doing heat-generated styles to your hair too much during this weather. You should wear hats to protect your hair, as well as your head. Wear a satin scarf underneath the hat to protect your hair from the hat's harsh fabrics that can cause friction, if the hat isn't already lined.

In the summer, the sun and humidity can be just as harsh for your hair (especially your ends), so try these tips:

Avoid washing your hair daily, and avoid using harsh shampoos (really should be year-round). The chlorine in swimming pools can be very drying for the hair. Try wetting the hair before going in the pool and even adding conditioner or shea butter if wearing a cap, so your hair doesn't absorb as much of the chlorine water as if it was dry. Then afterwards, use a mild shampoo to wash out the chlorine. Deep condition often. Sun damage can be harsh to the hair – if you're going to be out all day, use a lined straw hat to protect your hair from the sun (incorporate a loose satin scarf underneath if not lined, so the scalp can still breathe). Note: Avoid tight-fitting caps and any headwear that will make you sweat; it promotes bacteria, fungus, and hair loss. Wear plenty of braids, twists, and buns to avoid frizzy hair, and try to stay away from any kind of chemical influences (like dyes) or any product that has alcohol in it. If you don't normally use natural products, try switching just for the summer months. For frizzy hair, use jojoba oil to treat your strands throughout the day, or even as an overnight treatment. It works great on frizzy and dry hair. Try to keep split ends at bay by trimming the hair often. Above all, drink plenty of water. Continue to hydrate yourself throughout the day, and decrease your alcohol intake.

Caring for Children's Natural Hair

I have a cousin that recently went natural and when she first cut off her hair, it was late in the day and she wanted to wash it. I coincidentally didn't have any shampoo, so we went to the supermarket to try to find something that wouldn't be harmful to her newly-cut natural hair.

After reading 10 shampoo bottles that had sodium laureth sulfate, I instinctively went for the baby shampoo, because in my mind, we buy baby shampoo because its ingredients are simpler and gentler for the baby, right? To my surprise, they all had it as well, along with a lot of other undesirable things. Wow.

So what do we do for young children? As far as washing and conditioning, I would suggest going for something natural, for the same reasons adults go for something natural: it's safer and less harsh for the hair. If our hair can't take it well, I can only imagine young children. But for a baby, let's take it a step further: there are things because of our habits, lifestyles and age that a baby will not need, so when you think of a baby's hair, think of buying something with the simplest ingredients you can find. A baby does not need anything strong to be bathed with or to wash their hair, so the simplest baby shampoo will do the job.

Like with our hair, babies' delicate strands do not fare well with rubbing on the material of a pillow or on cotton, and oftentimes we see the baldness around the sides and back of the head (coincidentally, the same places that the hair rubs). We have come to know this as a normal process in babies' hair growth, but people who do preventative maintenance for this problem have definitely seen great results. Many people find it difficult to wrap something on a baby's head that will stay put, so an option would be to line a soft, thin, baby's hat (so it's not too hot) with satin on the inside for when they're sleeping. There's also the method of securing satin on the top of the mattress tightly (to prevent any suffocation) where the baby's head rests, or covering the baby's pillow (tightly again) with satin, if you have a baby that stays on his/her pillow.

Some mothers use Vaseline on their baby's heads to slick it down and make the curls look shiny. Petroleum Jelly is not good for the hair or the scalp, and should not be used on you or your baby's hair.

Young girls' hair, like your hair, needs moisture, soft hands, and protective styles. Because children play a lot, are on the floor, and get into a lot of things, protective styles should be implemented most of the time, with leaving the hair out only for special occasions. Rubber bands or even coated bands are definitely not something to be used in a young girl's hair; because the hair is so delicate, oftentimes the hair pulls right out of the scalp, and causes hair loss along the line.

For children with thick hair and tender scalps, please look into a detangler and a creamy leave-in to help soften the curls and coat the shaft, for less dry and/or coarse hair. Wash hair in braided sections to avoid having to detangle as much after washing, and detangle while the conditioner or leave-in is in the damp hair, never dry.

Some suggestions: Taiykel Afro Detangler appears to have great results for detangling and softening children's Type 4 hair; Taliah Waajid has an herbal comb out conditioner for children's Type 3 and 4 hair with great results; and if your child has a finer grade of hair, but the hair is frizzy and hard to manage, The Mixed Chicks line has been raved about for the results in children's Type 2 and 3 hair. These are just starting points, I'm sure there are many more. Please do your research and look for something for your child's hair type.

Section 2: The Endless Possibilities with Natural Hair

I really wanted this section of the book to be in full color, but it would have driven up the cost of the book significantly, and in the end, I wanted the book to be affordable. So to make up for this shortcoming, I have made this part of the book available on electronic download for anyone who has bought a copy, in full color. Simply go to the website, reclaimnaturalbeauty.com, go to the members only section, type in the ISBN number (found on the back of the book, no spaces or dashes) as the password, and you can download this entire section in full color.

Natural Hair Testimonials

The following are a handful of the submissions I received that I wanted to share. These ladies are a broad variety of beautiful, natural girls with their own story to tell about why they became natural. They come from all walks of life, all ages, numerous backgrounds, and varying timeframes of how long they've been natural.

These ladies have learned to appreciate their natural hair, and are on their way to achieving long, strong, beautiful hair (if they're not already there).

Enjoy.

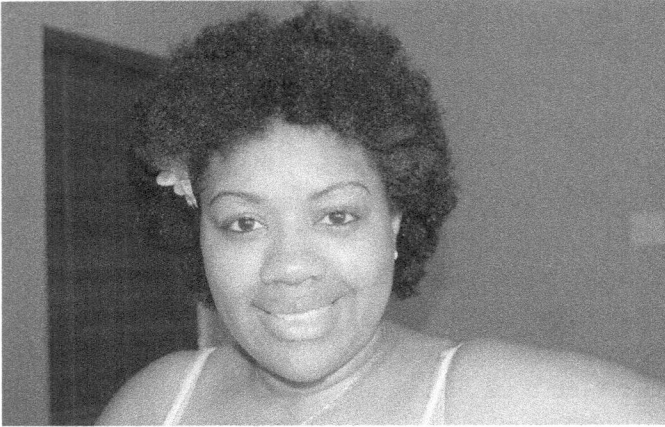

Anna L.
P. Pines, FL
Hair Type: 4A
Natural for:
8 mths

When my sister suggested that I go natural, I laughed hysterically. I said my hair was too nappy; there was no way I could go without a perm. Then a year ago, I gave myself a perm that went horribly wrong. When I washed it out, handfuls of my hair went with it. It was then that I decided to "entertain" the idea of going natural. I reasoned it couldn't get any worse. Once I passed the 6-month mark, there was no going back. What made this attempt different from the others was I knew this time I wouldn't be able to remain natural unless I learned how to take care of my hair. The first thing that I learned was that I knew absolutely nothing about my hair. Everything about maintaining natural hair was different from processed hair. Even the way I wash my hair is different. I tried several products until I found ones that were compatible with my hair. Going natural takes a lot of planning, sacrifice & dedication. One thing I will say, however, is that I'll never go back to perms. My hair hasn't been this thick and healthy since I was a child. Did I mention how beautiful my natural hair is?

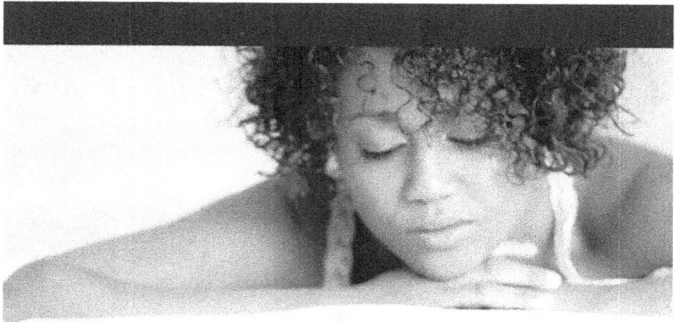

Fiamma S.
Miami, FL
Hair Type: 3B
Natural For:
Most of my life

One of my earliest memories is my mother beating my head up with the comb because it was so thick and long. I disliked my hair so much, when I came of age to handle it on my own, I just slicked it back every day. When I turned 18, I chopped it off. It took about 4 yrs to get it back to the length of my youth. Then I came to embrace the big hair God gave me. But the longer it got, the thicker it became. So thick, it took 10 mins to detangle in the shower. So my stylist gave me the idea to do a reverse curl treatment. First wash afterwards, my hair began to fall out in chunks. More on the 2nd wash. I ran back to the salon and they said they would do the Brazilian treatment to straighten my hair until it grew back to a decent length. They assured me that my curls would come back – they never did. The 2 treatments ruined my hair. I had to chop it off again – this time, not by choice. It's been app. 2 years & my hair is still short (because it works for me) & process free. I appreciate my hair more than I ever have. I will never again alter the natural beauty that was given to me at birth.

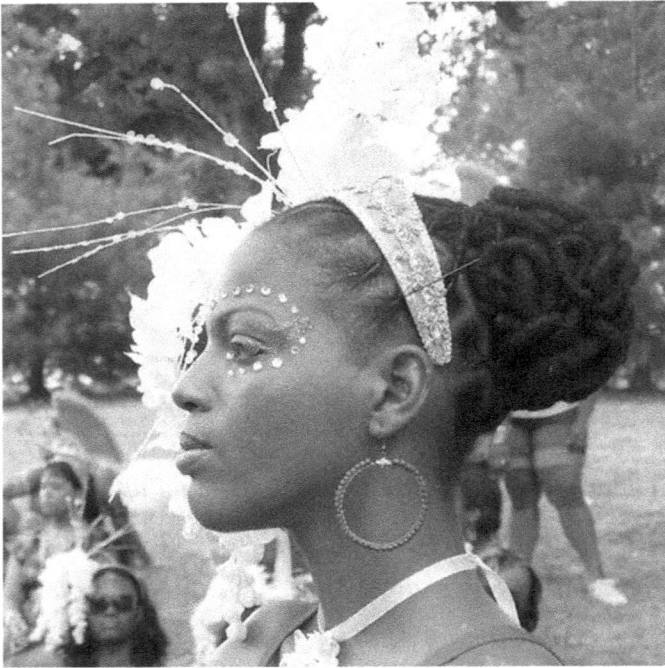

Name: **Amoy F.**
Trinidad, WI
Hair type: Unknown
Natural for: 4 yrs

The love for natural hair doesn't necessarily stem from the urge and longing to embrace your roots. It has now become a lifestyle decision. For years I have lived with a perm, holding on to a love for locks. As I matured in society, I realized there was a stigma placed on locks. A stigma I could not avoid if I had to choose my career path.

As the modern man began to accept the authenticity of African heritage in the workplace, locks became more accepted. I made the decision to choose my love for locks and battle for my place in the workforce. I went all natural on December 2, 2006. It requires a certain level of commitment. That commitment to nurture your hair and let it grow: the use of natural products, steaming, grooming and pampering. I believe people see you before they get to know you. Your hair is your beauty and needs to reflect that you are beautiful by always looking its best. I pay careful attention to it without leaning towards appearing vain and self-consumed. I wash, twist and restyle on a regular basis (every two weeks) with the attempt of always maintaining a professional, well-groomed appearance. You are constantly being watched, even when you are not aware. Judgments are constantly tossed at you because of your appearance. I am enjoying letting my natural beauty shine through!

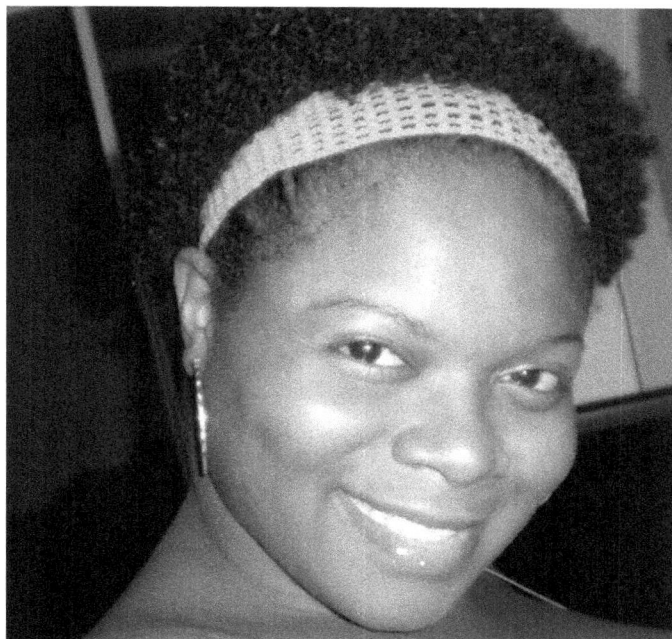

Camille T.
Miami, FL
Hair Type: 4A
Natural For:
3 mths

The last time I saw my natural hair, I was 8 years old, and I didn't remember what my natural hair even looked like. Even when I had new growth, I still didn't know, I just figured that's how everyone's hair looked: dry and hard. For years I'd been perming it, and I finally came to my breaking point. Thanksgiving of 2009 was the last time I had a perm, and I'd been holding on to my idea of "good hair" for six months. On June 13, 2010, I made the decision to cut my relaxed hair off. It was half the length of my index finger. It was the most liberating experience. Emotionally, I was free from dry, brittle, lifeless hair and discovered the real truth behind having beautiful, natural hair. It's been 3 months, and I still don't regret my decision to go natural. Some of the styles that I have experimented with my short hair turned out to be quite sexy. And today I am continuing my quest in achieving and enjoying my beautiful locs. A year from now, I'm looking forward to having long, lustrous, natural hair!

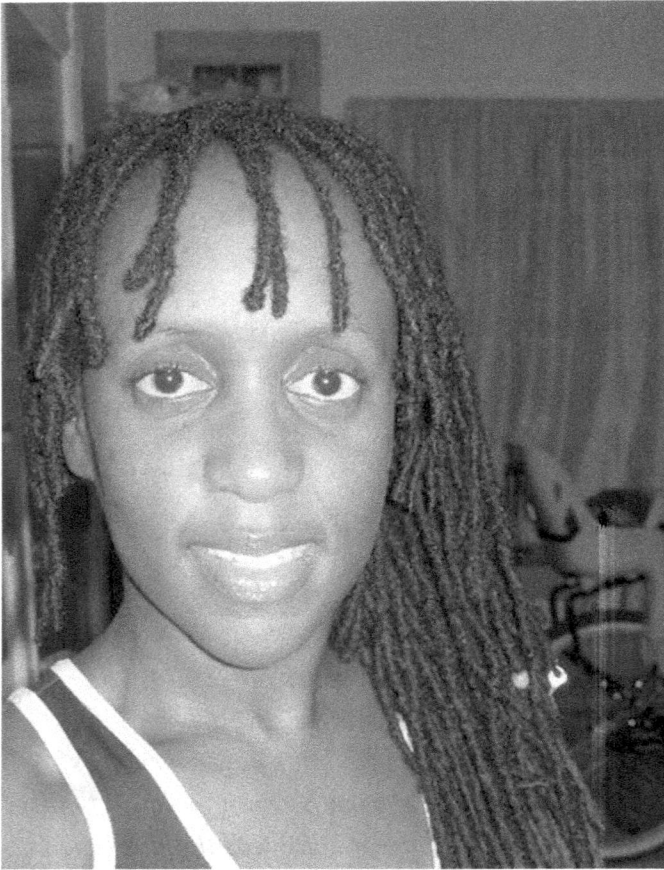

Nicole Neda P.
DC Metro area
Natural for:
12 yrs

Back in 1998, I decided to go natural, because I simply wanted to stop depending on the creamy "crack" they call a relaxer. It was beginning to break my hair and it was time to reverse the damage it caused. I sported an afro for the first few months, then I began the process of locking my hair. I had locks for over 10 years, until I thought I missed combing my hair. After less than a year, I realized I didn't like combing my hair anymore, lol. Now I'm regrowing my locks again and love them! :)

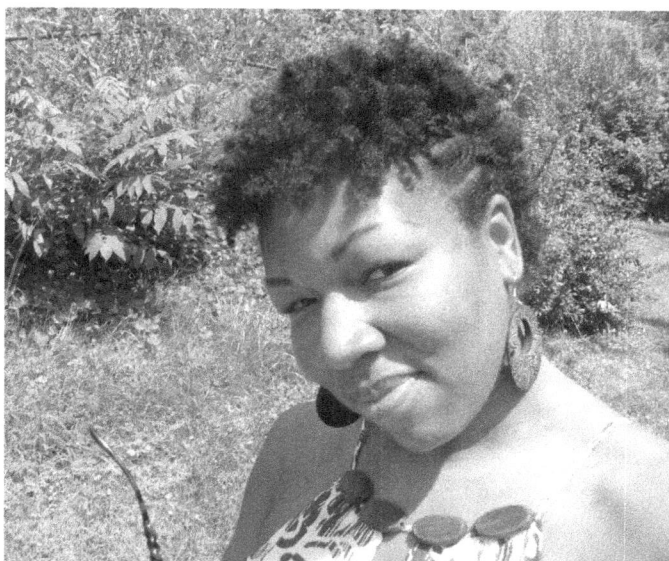

Stacy L.
Lexington, KY
Hair type:
Unknown
Natural for:
3 mths

I was inspired to go natural because of my daughter who has been natural for over 2 years. I was on the fence for a while and not totally committed, so before I actually made a final decision to transition, I stretched my relaxer for about 4 months, getting my roots & edges flat ironed during that time. After seeing the movie "Good Hair" and watching a relaxer eat through a Coke can, that was when I made the decision that I was going natural for sure. I planned to transition for one year, but grew tired of dealing with two textures. My actual transition time was just shy of 9 months. I cut my relaxer off slowly over that time and got rid of the last of the relaxed ends on May 20, 2010. I've been natural for just over 3 months now and I love it!

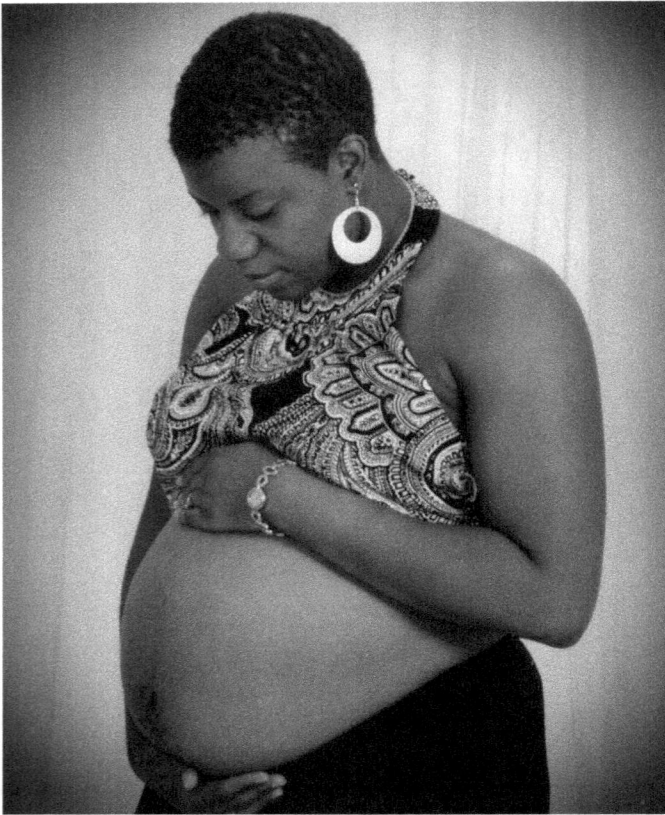

Chely T.

Ft Lauderdale, FL

Hair Type: Unknown

Ntrl for: 5+ yrs

Having dealt with an excessive sweating problem for years and being unable to maintain certain styles because of this, I decided to go natural and have never looked back. For the last 4 years I had locks which I loved, but felt a need for a change and went right back to what I like to call "the nothing to hide look." This style is comfortable, easily manageable, and clean; it still requires some care though. I use natural products which include moisturizers, pomades and some curl crèmes. Depending upon the length, I range from buzz to mini fro and I change colors depending upon what mood I'm in; it's fun, it's easy and it's bold. I must mention recently I had a very young man say, "You know you're beautiful if you can pull that off." I love it! Enjoy your personal discovery and remember that your approval is the only one that counts.

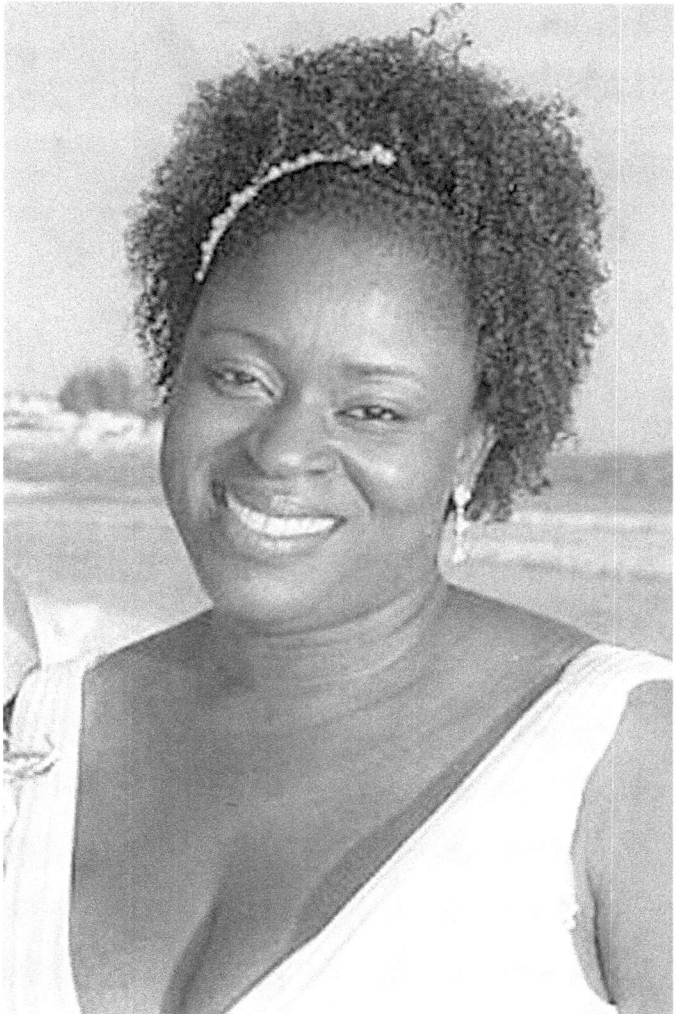

Shelley A.
St. Georges,
Grenada
Hair Type: 4A
Natural for: 6 yrs

Beauty is knowing who you are and loving it. Being natural for 6 years has been a challenge at times, but with gained knowledge and support of others, it has been an enjoyable one. I have learned over the years that I am beautiful, regardless of the kinks in my hair.

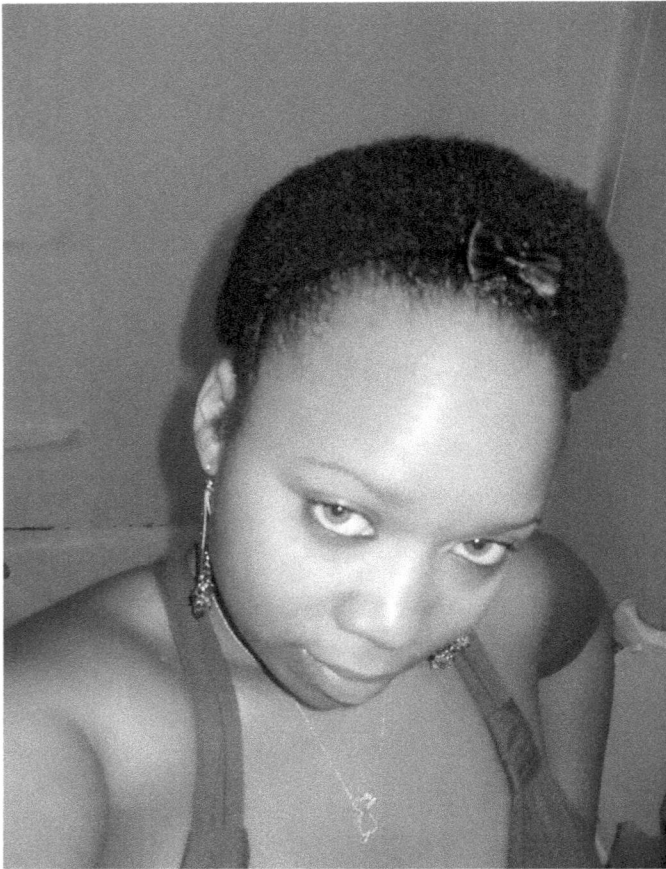

Alishia R.
Merrillville, IN
Hair type: (5C, LOL), I think maybe 3A-3B
Natural for: 11 mths and ♥ing it...

I went natural after being inspired by several youtube videos! I love every minute of my natural hair and I have never felt soooooo beautiful as I do now. Being natural is a bold statement that says "I am okay with who I naturally am."

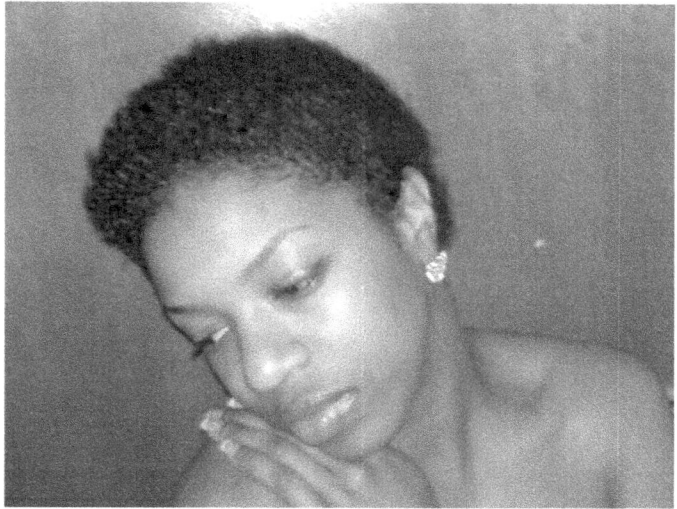

Virgillette A.
Milwaukee, WI
Hair Type: 4A/B
Natural for:
2.5 mths

Accepting my natural texture and self-love are almost parallel to one another in my journey. It has allowed me to be more open-minded, not just with hair, but people! Natural hair speaks for itself. As natural black women, we have a VARIETY of curly and kinky textures and I love that! It's about time that more women embrace this journey as well.

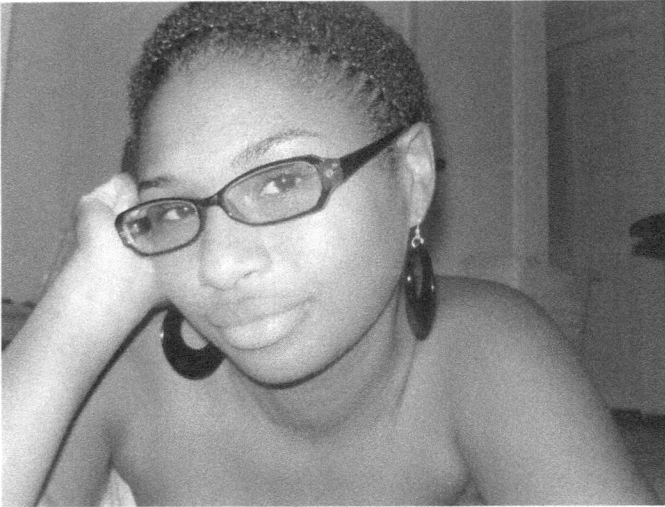

Shantavia C.
Jacksonville, FL
Hair Type:
3C/4A
Natural for:
1 mth

I think going natural was one of the greatest decisions I have made in my life. I was in love with MY Hair from the moment I did my big chop. My hair is strong, healthy and very versatile. Also contrary to belief, it's very manageable and low maintenance. I can literally wash and go. With my natural hair, I can have my cake and eat it too.

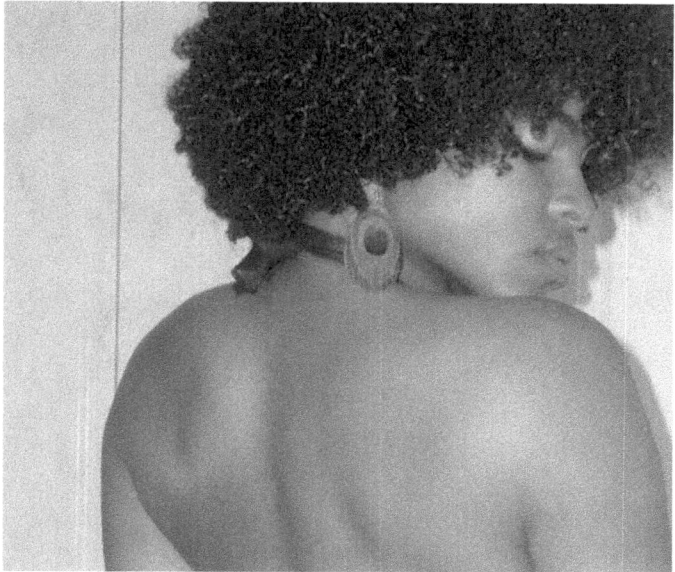

Sherica P.

Hollywood, FL

Hair Type: Not sure

Natural For: My whole life!

My mommy never permed me or my sister's hair. She felt that it was way too permanent and damaging to the hair and if we wanted to take the path to relaxed hair, it had to be when we were old enough to make our own decisions, but it wouldn't be by her. By the time we finally did come of age, we had already gotten use to styling, caring for, and loving our natural tresses. Mama truly knows best!

I've always enjoyed styling and caring for my hair and loved how it made me stand out alongside my personality. In high school, I experimented with lots of different styles that included braids and twists (mostly protective styling). When I got to college, I not only learned how care for my hair in a healthier manner, but I also got into fashion as well. Next year I start taking pre-med courses at USF in Tampa Fl. and intend on taking my "afro chic" look with me! I can't wait! Right now I am the co-owner of the Shatterproof Glass Dolls blogsite and soon to be website, with my just as natural and equally fabulous big sister, Taneica!

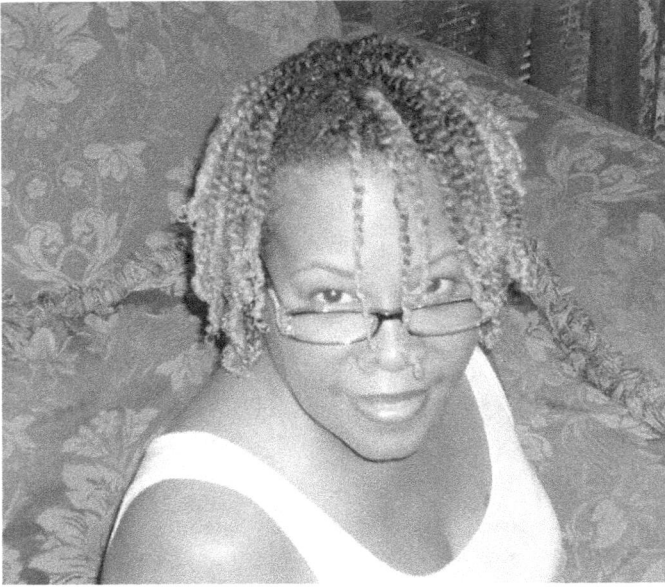

Raenel S.
Dallas, TX
Hair Type: 3C
Natural for: 3 yrs

I initially went natural because I had to either give up my perm or my color because my hair couldn't take both anymore. Now the longer I'm natural, the more I know I made the right decision. I love the God-given hair that I was blessed with and for all my sistas out there that are still addicted to the "creamy crack," come on over to the real side and celebrate the beautiful, black, and natural Queens we were all meant to be!

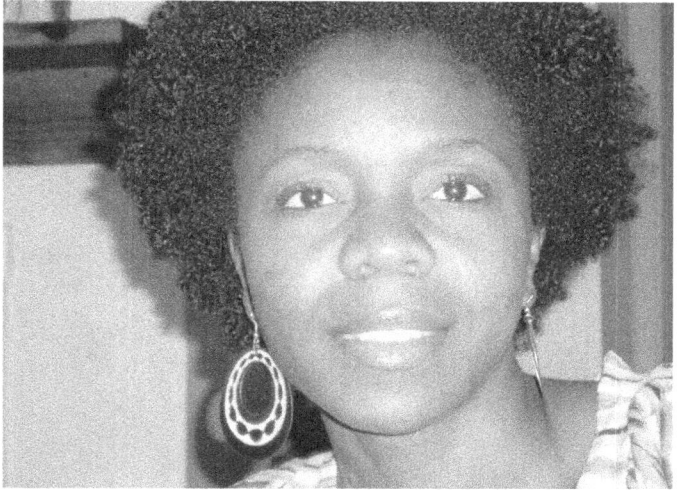

Zenobia J.
Tunica, MS
Hair Type: 4A
Natural for: 2 yrs

My decision to go natural was so much deeper than hair. It uncovered who I really am inside. It was hard to accept the new me, but now I am in love with God's creation and a mouthpiece for natural sisters everywhere.

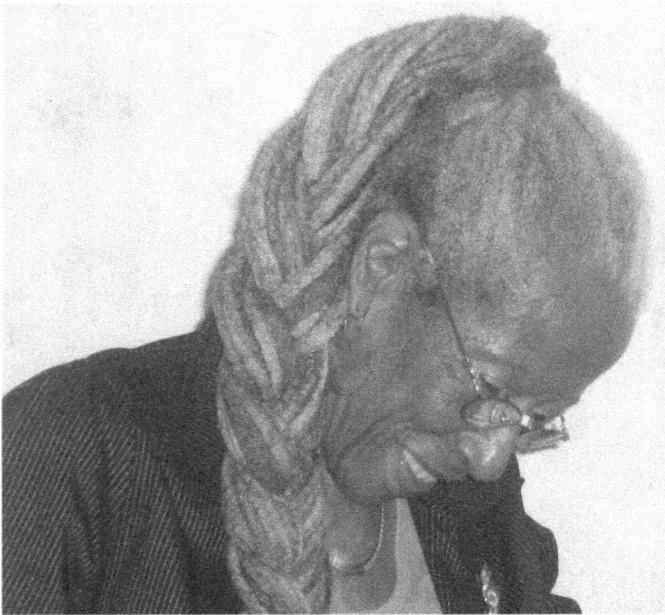

Peggye M.
San Antonio, TX
Hair Type: 4A,
B, and/or C
Natural for: 16
yrs (locks
14 yrs)

I received a diagnosis of liver disease, with the need for a liver trans-
plant anticipated. I decided to do the "Big Cut" on my dyed and
processed hair immediately. I vowed to cease the use of heat and
chemicals in my hair to reduce the loss that might come with surgery
(anesthesia) and medications.

I had been "natural" a couple of years when I took a vacation to Ja-
maica. While there, a local friend put my hair up in "Nubian Twists."
I had picked a photo of Blair Underwood on the cover of an Essence
Magazine to replicate.

Finding no one in San Antonio to maintain the style, on my return, I
started doing my own hair. I have done so since then and never looked
back. My hair is now at the length where I have to take care, trying to
avoid sitting on it.

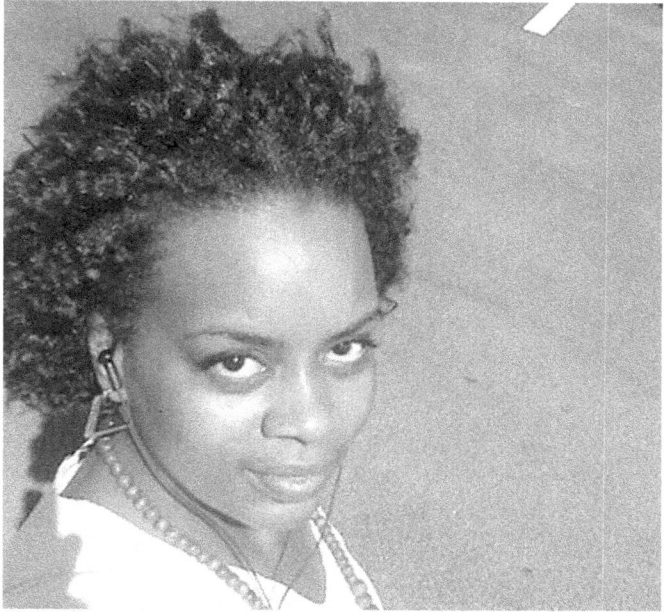

Hope B.

Pompano Bch, FL

Hair Type: Unknown

Natural for: 16 mths this time around; I wore locks for 8 years from 1999 to 2007

I had a tragic event occur in my personal life last year and just decided to make some changes inside and out. So I sat in the mirror with scissors and a comb and cut off all my relaxed hair, and what was left almost gave my husband a heart attack. I looked like a sad little boy :-) but I felt really free. Since then, I have been growing and loving my hair and expanding the product line that I use.

I feel confident, pretty, and versatile. When I want to go straight, I can go straight, and when I want to be curly I can be curly. I missed out on that having locks. My hair texture is a bit difficult sometimes, but I always find a way to make it work. I also want to mention that I have been noticing more and more black women in TV commercials with natural hair than ever before. Looks nice!

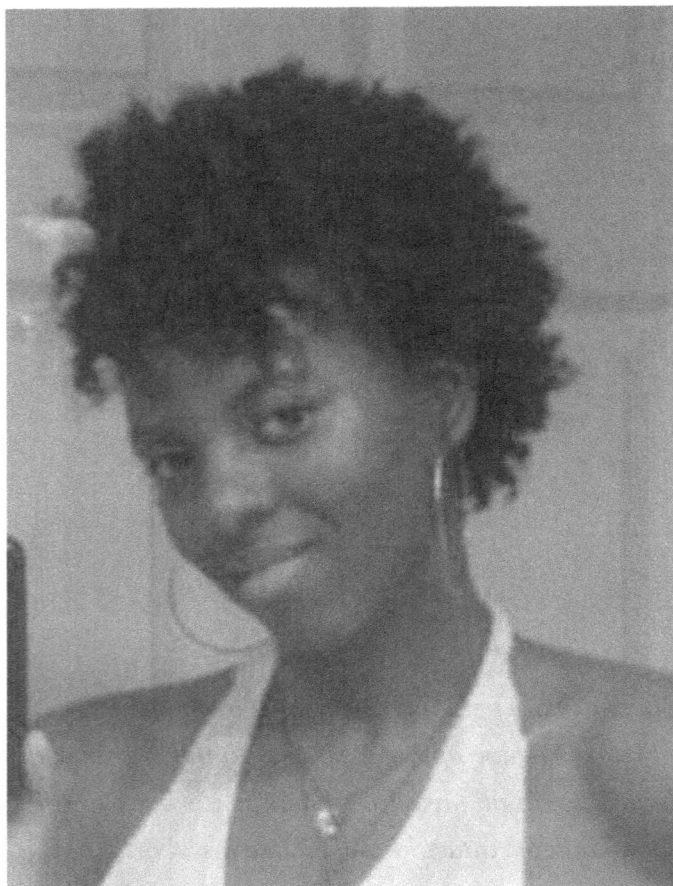

Name: **Asya W.**
Atlanta, GA
Hair Type: 4B
Natural for:
7 mths

The best thing that I have done for my hair is put together a good hair regimen. Do not expect to have it down pact the first week you go natural, it has taken me about six months to really find products that work and techniques I like. Be patient, persistent, and gentle.

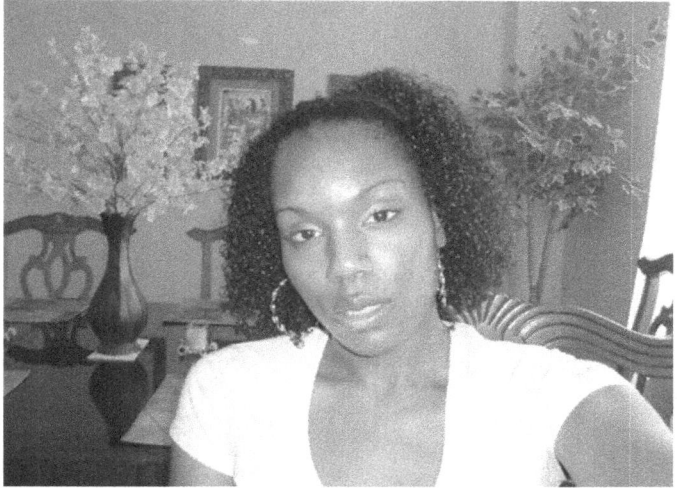

Antoinette R.
Jacksonville, FL
Hair Type:
Unknown
Natural for: 4 yrs

As a child, I always wanted to go natural. I had my first relaxer at age 4. In the beginning of my first three years, it was challenging, since I

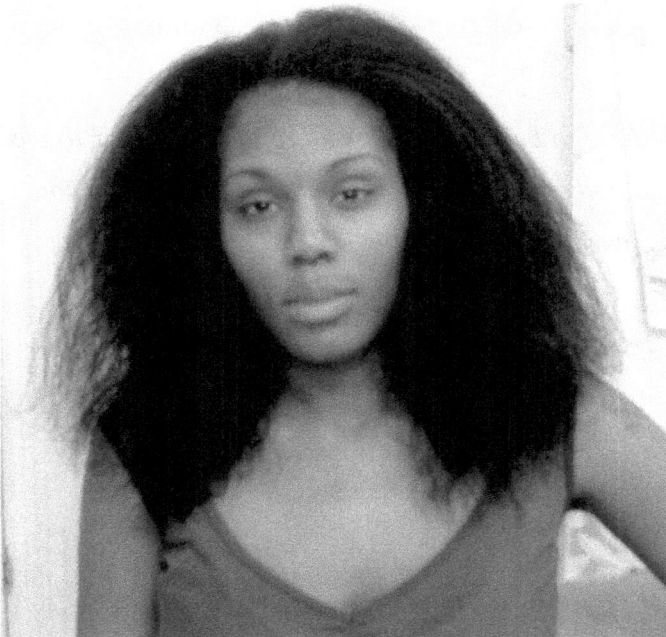

didn't know much about natural hair or what products to use.

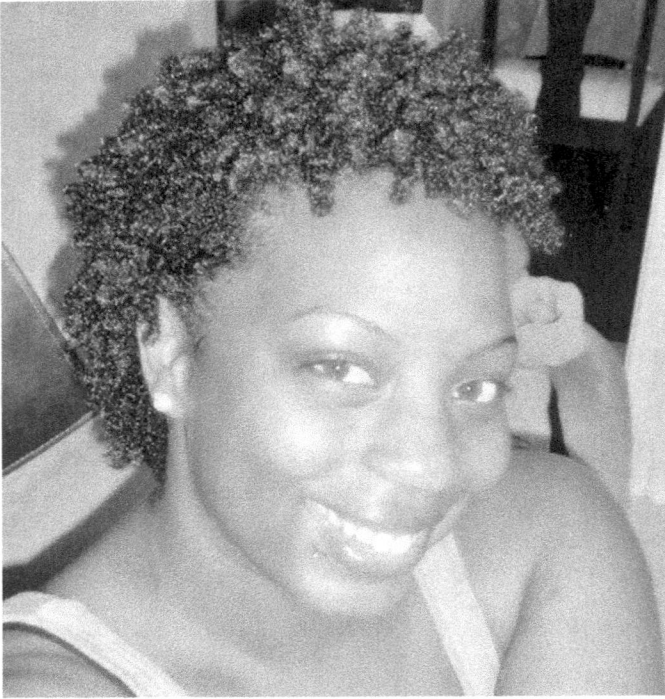

Lashanita M.
Little Rock, AR
Hair Type:
4A/4B
Natural for:
8 mths

Natural hair is something to be proud of. It's more than just hair to me, it's about being proud and comfortable with who you are. This is you, stripped down for the world to see and it is BEAUTIFUL.

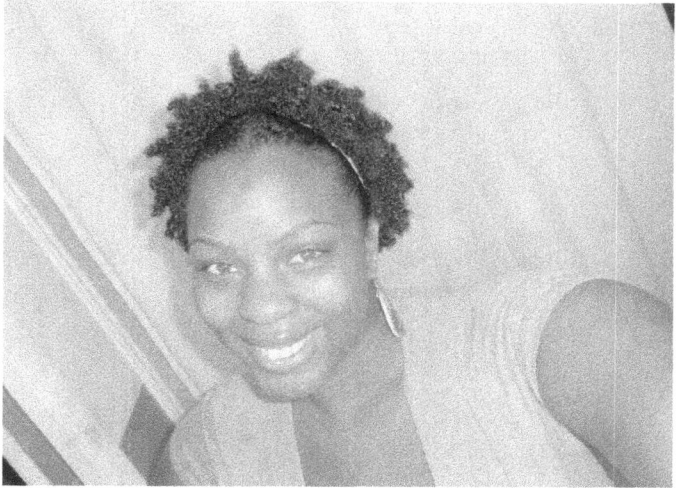

Tashanita M.
Little Rock, AR
Hair Type:
4A/4B
Natural for:
8 mths

Deciding to go natural was one of the best decisions I've ever made. I take such pride in my tresses. Whether I'm wearing it twisted up, picked out, or just letting it "do its own thing," I love it! I couldn't be happier. It's so me!

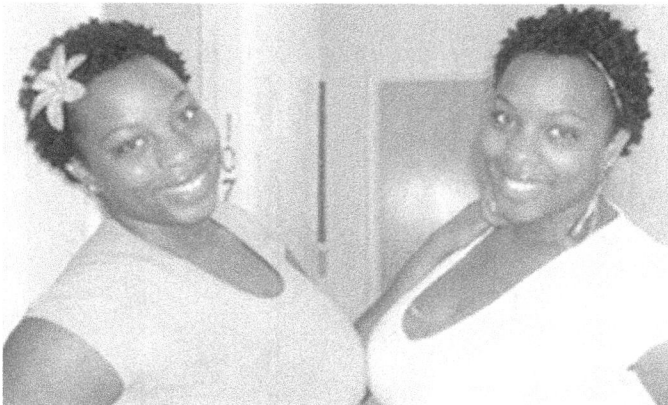

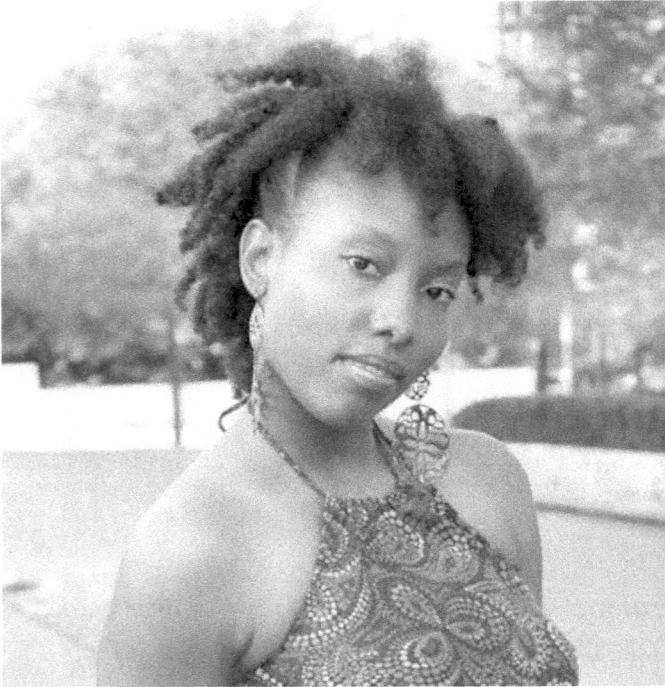

Natasha B.

Chicago, IL

Hair Type:
I really do not
know, it is thick
and tightly coiled

Natural for: 1 yr
and 3 mths

*This is my second time transitioning, I finally stuck to my plan this time
and transitioned for a year. I did my big chop in '09. I can honestly say
that I love my hair even more now, so goodbye to perms forever.*

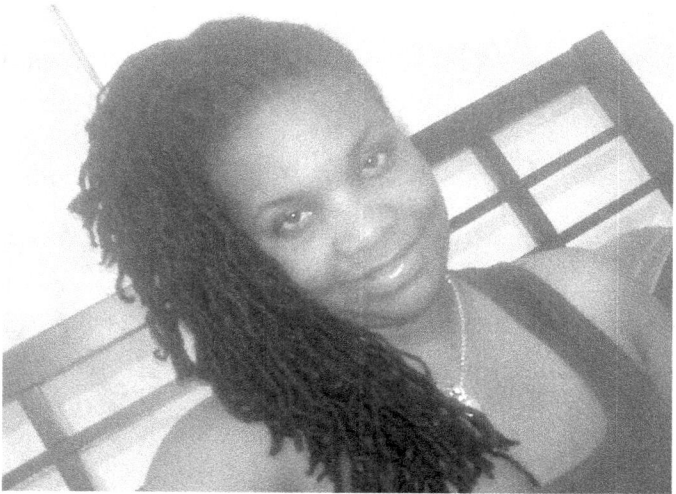

Zorana G.
Miami, FL
Hair type:
Unknown
Natural for: 7 yrs

I decided to go natural because perming my thick lengthy hair became a nightmare; each time it burned and left my scalp sore. With that, I decided to begin my natural journey! I love my beautiful hair!

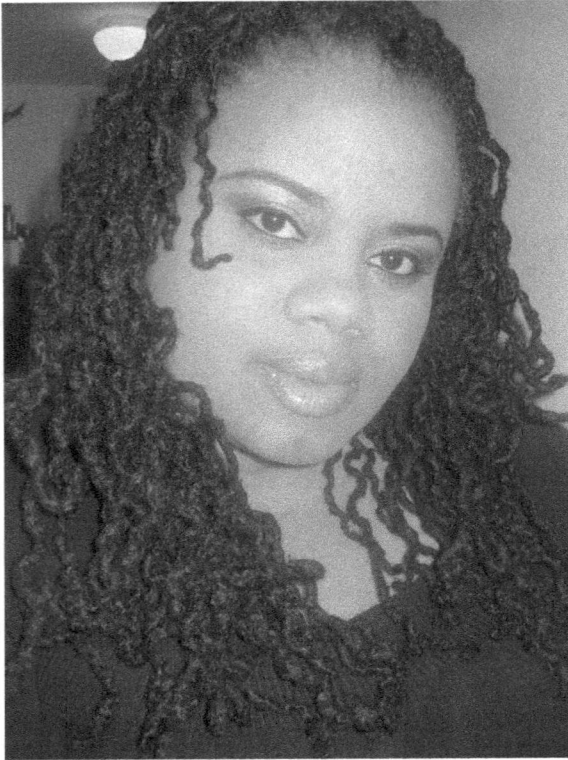

Shirley A.
Boynton Bch, FL
Hair Type:
Unknown
Natural for: 6 yrs

I always wanted to be natural, but it took me a while to finally make the decision. Working in Corporate America, I wasn't sure I'd be able to look professional and wasn't sure how I'd react to the stares. But living in Florida, the humidity caused me to relax my hair monthly (which I knew wasn't healthy). So one day I had enough and stopped at a barbershop and ask the barber to cut it all off. After about 10 min of arguing with him, he finally did it. I left the shop feeling FREE (literally). I wore it in a short buzz cut for about six months. Soon afterwards I set an appointment with a loctician because I knew locking my hair was my ultimate goal. I decided to let my hair grow and then with my hair at about 4-5" long, she double strand twisted it and eventually, my hair started locking (it took a year or so to lock, it depends on your hair type). I haven't looked back since. I absolutely love my locs... all I do is add some olive oil to it weekly and use Organic Root Stimulator products (it's very low maintenance, I don't even own a comb or brush). I plan on being "Naptural" forever...

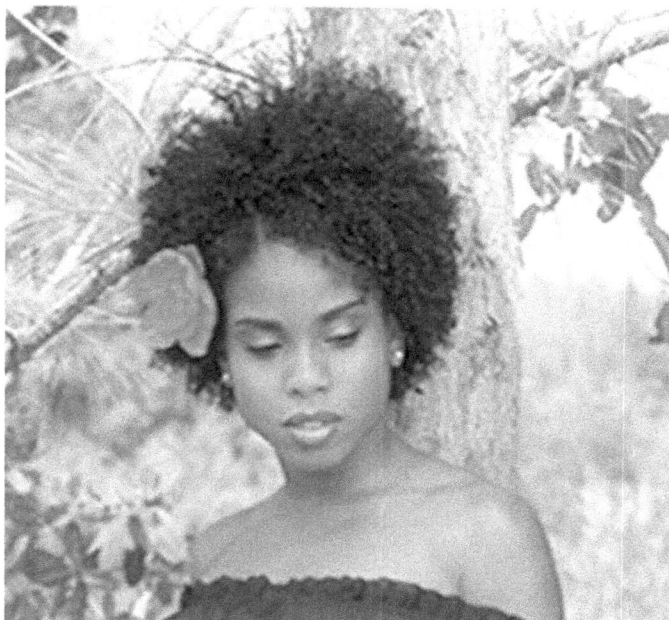

Meliana A.

Ft Lauderdale, FL

Hair Type: Unknown

Natural for: 12 yrs

I've had pretty thick hair all my life and relaxing it was causing dryness and shedding. Right out of high school, I decided I had no other choice but to go natural if I wanted my hair to be healthy again. It's been over 10 years now, and my chemical-free hair is still turning heads. Natural hair is very versatile. I can wear it in an afro, braid styles or straighten it for a new look. This is definitely the best decision I made for my hair, and my hair thanks me every day.

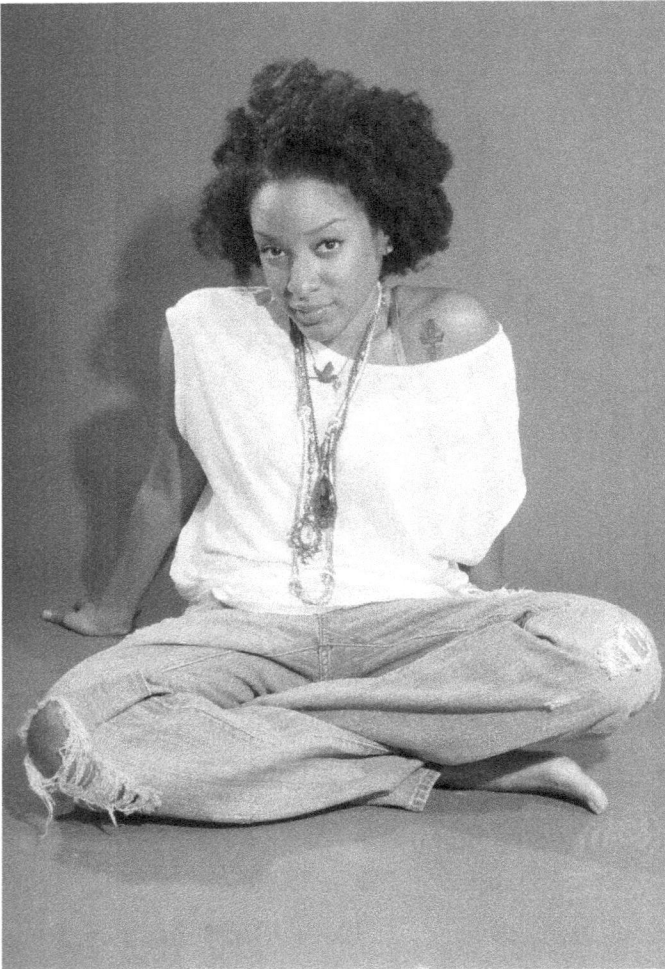

Nia D.
Miramar, FL
Hair Type:
Unknown
Natural for: 2 yrs

Shaving off my hair was very traumatizing. I cried for two days, but it turned out to be a liberating experience. I have a newfound freedom, no longer bound by a box of chemical relaxer. I absolutely love my hair and the men dig it a lot too, lol.

144

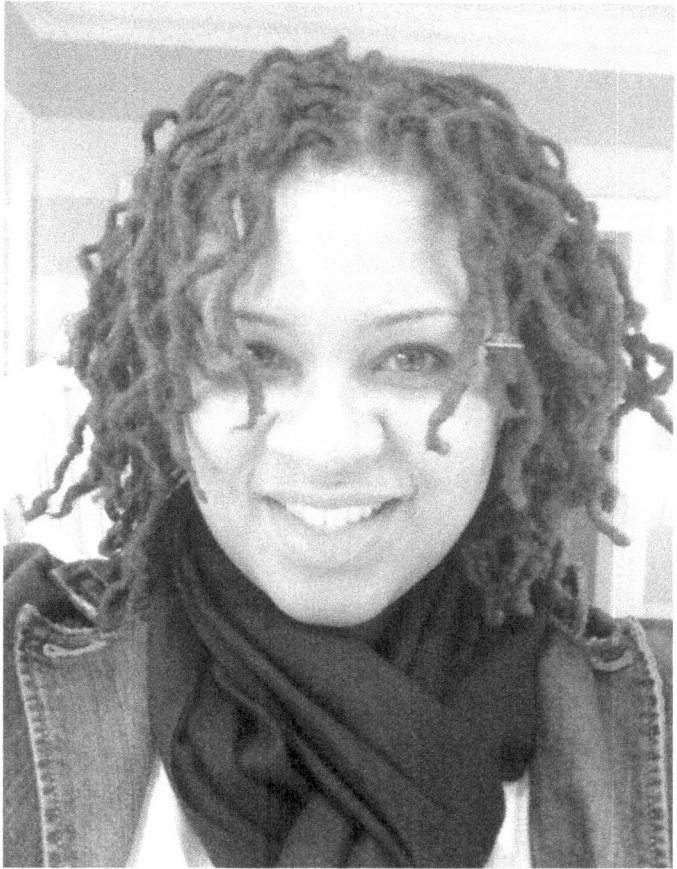

Nikki H.

Huntington Sta, NY

Hair Type: 3C

Natural for: 2 yrs

I was 22 when I first went natural. I loved wearing the double strand twist! In 1997, I locked my hair for the first time! I grew my locks until the winter of '01. I cut my hair because I felt I needed a change… So the fastest thing to change was my hair! I am now sorry that I did that! I tried to go back to the relaxer, but my scalp was entirely too sensitive.

For a while I rocked the fro'. However, the fro was too high maintenance for me and I am now back to my dreads, with a second birth date of February 08'

I love and I will always stay natural!!!!!!

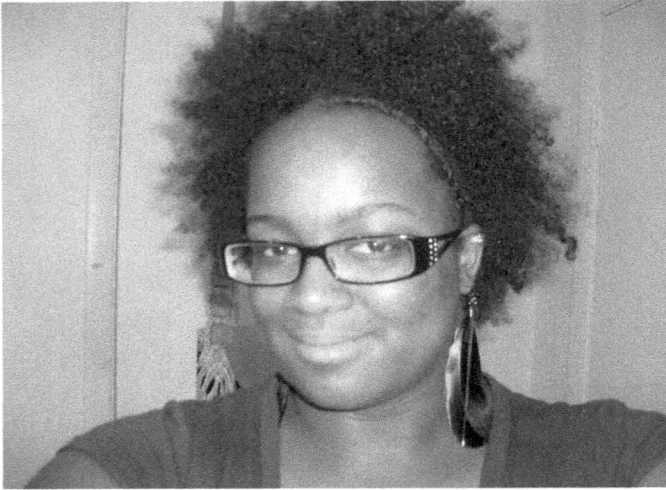

Name: **Ashlee L.**
Virginia Bch, VA
Hair type: 3C
Natural for:
6 mths

After the first failed attempt to go natural, I was very destined and determined to go all the way. When I finally "big chopped," I was not only liberated, but I had fallen in love with my hair. Although I've had ups and downs with my new hair, I have a tremendous amount of support from family, friends and patience from God. I can truly say that I'm very blessed with "good hair." To those sisters and brothers who are about to give up, I say don't, because you're defeating the purpose and losing the fight. Keep holding on, have patience, and there is support all around you. God bless! And remember, be happy that you are nappy!

Easy, Everyday Natural Styles

Braid outs, twist outs, Bantu knot outs

Braid outs and twist outs are basically the process of braiding or two-strand twisting the hair overnight (or for several hours, or days), then loosening out the braids or twists (without combing it out), separating the strands (not much, maybe in two or three sections) and wearing the style with the wave, crimp, or curl that the braids or twists have left in your hair. Some people will curl the ends with small rods, but I don't do this. The bigger the braids or twists, the larger the waves, crimps or curls will be in your hair. I personally don't like to do the sections too small; I like them to be medium to big in size, so that the curls or waves are bigger and more defined in my hair. But I have seen some people do them small and they look awesome. I personally think it will have to do with what size curls or waves you're starting with (your natural curl pattern). One thing to be aware of is how you part the hair when braiding or twisting it, because that's the parts you'll have when taking them out. I find that trying to make a part and moving the hair around in the opposite direction after taking out the braids or twists can be difficult, and can make the hair lose some of the definition it had. I love both braid outs and twist outs, but if I have to choose, I would say I'm more favorable to twist outs. Bantu knot outs are the idea of not two-strand twisting the hair, rather just taking the entire lock of hair and twisting it, then wrapping it around and around it into a Bantu knot (or Chinese Bump), then tucking in the ends, using a scrunchie to hold it or clipping it down so it stays knotted. The result when taken down is a very curly, bouncy, wavy style that is very beautiful. Same thing applies: the bigger the knots, the bigger the curls. I've done as little as two Bantu knots in my hair and the hair ended up with these huge waves. It just didn't last long, because my hair started to revert back to its natural curl pattern. A styling foam, crème or gel can help this. When taking any of the styles down, please be mindful of being soft and gentle, so that the hair doesn't frizz up and lose its definition. It is also helpful to put a little oil on your fingertips when taking the hair down to aid in preventing frizzing. Here is my take on them all:

Braid Outs, My Pros and Cons:

Braid outs, to me, offer you the ability to show off more of your hair's length than twist outs, because the braids keep your hair in a more taut state when braided. My favorite hairstyle for braids is cornrowing the front and single braiding or twisting the back. I have been doing that style since my hair has been natural; it's a cute style when your hair is short, and it's still great when your hair is long. My sister expanded on the style and cornrowed the front, then Bantu-knotted the back. It looks so cute. Another variation is to cornrow the front, and wear your braid outs or twist outs in the back. It immediately dresses up the style if you're going out, simply loosen out (take down) the braids in the back, split them and go.

Braid outs also last longer to me. The crimp style can stay in my hair for several days, whereas the twist outs (for me, anyway) can only last a few days. I think this is for the same reason – the braids are tighter and therefore stay longer when taken out.

The bigger braid outs (use fewer and fatter braids to achieve this style, as little as 6 braids for the entire head, depending on your length) or even big, cornrow braid outs (maybe 5 cornrows going back) can give you a beautiful wavy look. Very chic for going out.

Cornrow braids outs have more of a big curl (as opposed to a crimp or wave) than the single braids; plus you can wear the braids for a few days, then convert the style to the braid outs afterwards; so this is really two styles in one.

Con – Unlike twist outs, the braid outs don't look as natural (something your hair just normally looks like) as the twist outs. Because of this, I have to actually be in the mood to do braid outs; whereas the twist outs, it looks like it's my natural hair, while giving me a looser curl definition than my natural curls.

I like to keep my hair in a protective style, while maybe wearing it out during the weekend if I so choose. So for the single braids, when I braid my hair smaller to last for the week, I don't like the braid out style as much. It's not as defined in my hair as it would be if the braids were bigger. Therefore, single braid outs for me don't offer the "two style" bonus that I get with the twist outs; either I'm wearing the single braids, or I'm wearing my hair in big braids at night for the braid outs.

Twist Outs, My Pros and Cons:

- For me, the twist outs offer a more natural-looking style in the twists AND the twist out styles. The medium-sized twists give my hair such a neat look and they are very versatile to wear in almost any style I can do when my hair's loose. I wear this style often during the week; then later, I loosen the hair out (take it down) and leave the twist outs for the weekend. I love the way my hair curls in the twists, and it feels so soft, while staying moist. Then my curls look so defined when I take them out and wear the twist outs.

- The twists in my opinion are easier to do than the braids, and faster.

- BUT... I can put four braids in my hair and get a fierce, wavy style, but I cannot do the same for the twists, because they will come out while I'm sleeping, or just not maintain the twist out style for very long. I think once your hair reaches very long lengths, depending on your type of curl, this would no longer be a problem; but for now, if you want that big curly style, you have to do Bantu knots.

Some people do flat twists – the twist-equivalent of cornrows. Same concept of cornrowing by picking bits of hair up as you go applies to flat-twisting, only you now have two strands to work with instead of three. This method didn't stay in everyone's hair we tried it in. My cousin has 4A hair, but it is extremely soft and fine, so once we attempted to flat-twist her hair, it came right out (her hair is short though, only a few months natural). My hair is much thicker and not as fine, so it stays in my hair (even when it was short), but I don't achieve the same definition as I do with the single twists, so I really only do them to stretch out the hair, or to keep my twist outs overnight. I do think if I were to use something to set it with, it would stay longer; but as you all know by now, I'm not big on using those kinds of products.

Bantu Knot Outs, My Pros and Cons:

- As I said before, Bantu knot outs leave you with beautiful, curly, bouncy waves. You can wear the Bantu knots if you like, then wear the knot-out style. Some people get very creative in how they part the Bantu knots on their head, which results in a very beautiful style.

- My biggest complaint about Bantu knots, especially when your hair gets longer and the knots are bigger, is wearing them at night. Maybe I am just tender-headed, but they hurt, and are not comfortable for me at all. To sleep with them when your hair is shorter and you may need hairpins to keep them in place was not great for me either. I would rather put them in my hair early in the morning and leave them in all day, then wear the knot out for an evening style.

- Also, getting the ends to look good can be tricky if you can't get the knot to stay in place without hairpins or clips. The ideal Bantu knot look is achieved by wrapping the lock of hair all the way around on the outside of the knot (close to your scalp) until the entire thing is in the knot. But for some people/hair types, the knot starts to come loose, which results in some parts being defined when taken down, and others not. Clipping the ends down can also leave the hair with a little "bend" on the end of it, instead of a smooth natural-looking curl all the way down. Please keep this in mind when securing the knots. I've actually used small, soft scrunchies or coated rubber bands around the knots and that has worked for me without having to use hairpins or clips, so that's an option.

Wet versus Dry set:

- Like twist outs, when you braid the hair dry, it shows off more length in the end than when you braid them wet, but it still has less shrinkage than the twist outs either way. When braiding it dry, depending on your hair type, you may want to use some kind of setting lotion, like a twist and lock lotion, or even moisturize it really well with your moisturizer of choice and mist it well with water when braiding overnight.

- Wet set, however, in my opinion, results in a way more defined look, and lasts much longer. I can braid or twist my hair and leave it in all week when dry, then take it out and it will only last a few hours before my own curl pattern starts taking over. But if I do my twists or braids after washing my hair, even with big twists or braids, the definition of the style will last for days, to the point where it looks as if it's my natural curls. So for me, doing my twists wet are the way to go; curl definition is more important to me than the showing my length.

Now I wanted to experiment, because I realized that using the same method or products on different hair types does not always achieve the same results. So we tried twist outs, braid outs and Bantu knots on 3C, 4A (fine), and 4A/B (thick) hair, to see how it would come out.

My sister has 4A hair: Very thick, very dense, and not easy to manipulate. She wanted definition in her styles, but didn't want a hard, crunchy feeling. Her best results were with the Taliah Waajid Lock it Up Gel: It left her hair very defined, while still feeling very soft.

My cousin has very fine, yet very dense 4A hair. She does not need a lot of heavy products to keep her hair set, but because her curls are so small, she likes to use something to keep the different styles' looser curl definition: Her best results were with Kinky Curly Styling Spritz, adding a leave-in mix and Knot Today before the styling gel. She even had great results with just plain shea butter and big braids left overnight, or a wet set, letting it air dry.

My best results are always with a wet set. I usually don't use styling products; rather I condition my hair while it's wet with a leave-in mixture, seal it with some shea butter, and put medium-sized twists, braids, or knots in it. I then let it dry that way. When I'm ready to wear it out, I simply take out the twists, braids, etc. The one thing I will add is I usually put olive oil in my water mix that I mist my hair with, because it makes my hair look shiny and the color just pops. I love it.

After going to the natural hairdresser, we ALL had amazing results with the Nairobi Styling Foam. It kept the curl outs, twist outs, knot outs, rod sets – whatever style attempted – in place, stretched out, and without that crunchy or gel feeling.

This is the size of my natural curls, and how thick it is:

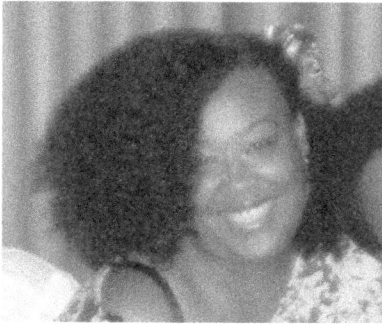

This however, is the size of twist outs I usually wear. I stay with twist outs very often:

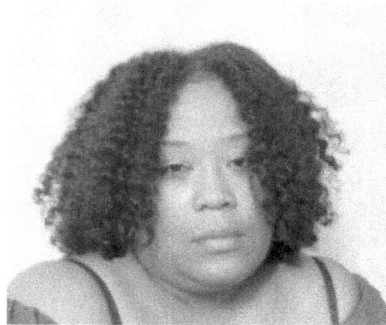

In the two pictures below, I was on vacation. I would just moisturize my hair at night and twist it in like 8 twists, take it out in the morning and style my hair.

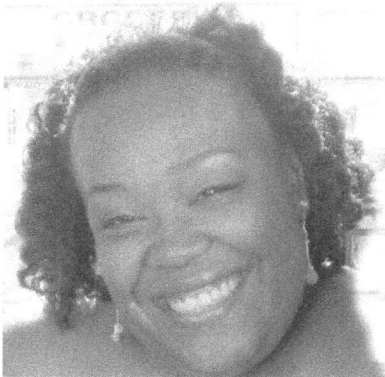

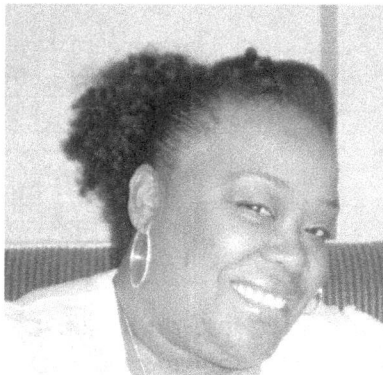

This is the style I got when I went to the natural hairdresser. Simone achieved this style by washing/conditioning my hair, parting it in small sections and adding the Nairobi Wrapp lotion to each strand, then two-strand twisting it. She then added medium-sized rollers to my hair, put a few braids on one side, and let me sleep in the rods. She used no heat, and the curls lasted for the week, even with me braiding my hair at night and adding my own oils and water to my hair:

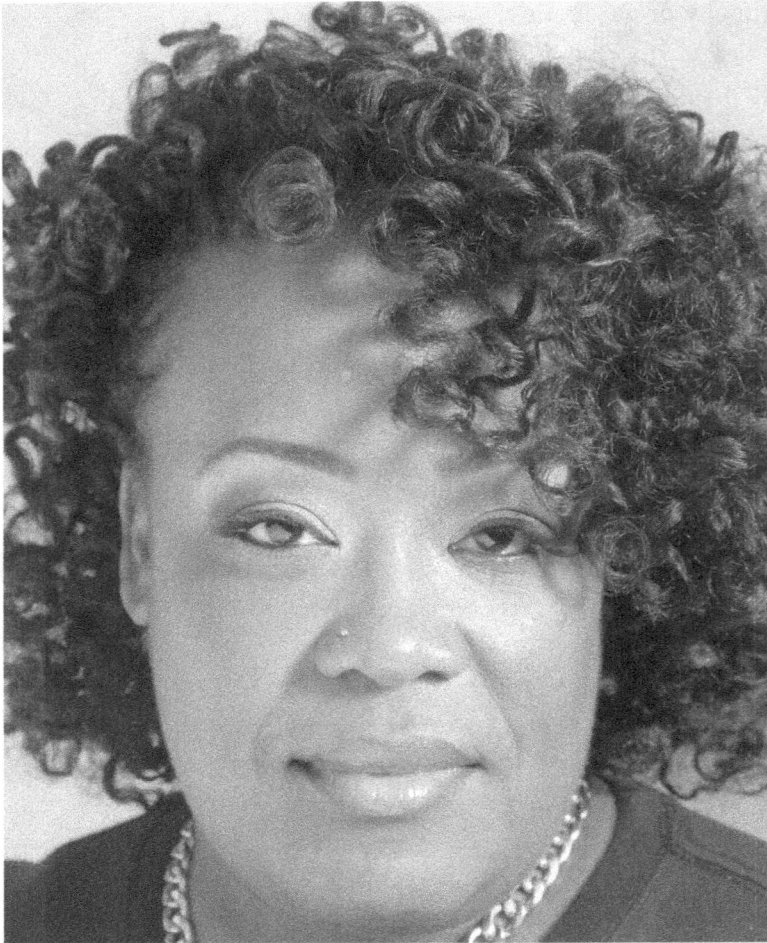

Hair: Simone Hylton, Natural Trendsetters, Makeup: Giselle Telesford. Photo: Justice Photography

Camille got a really edgy mohawk that I liked. Simone achieved this by washing/conditioning her hair and blow drying it to stretch it out, then braiding the sides and flat-twisting the middle in four big flat twists, using the Nairobi lotion. She slept in the flat-twists, and the next day after taking it out, the result were this:

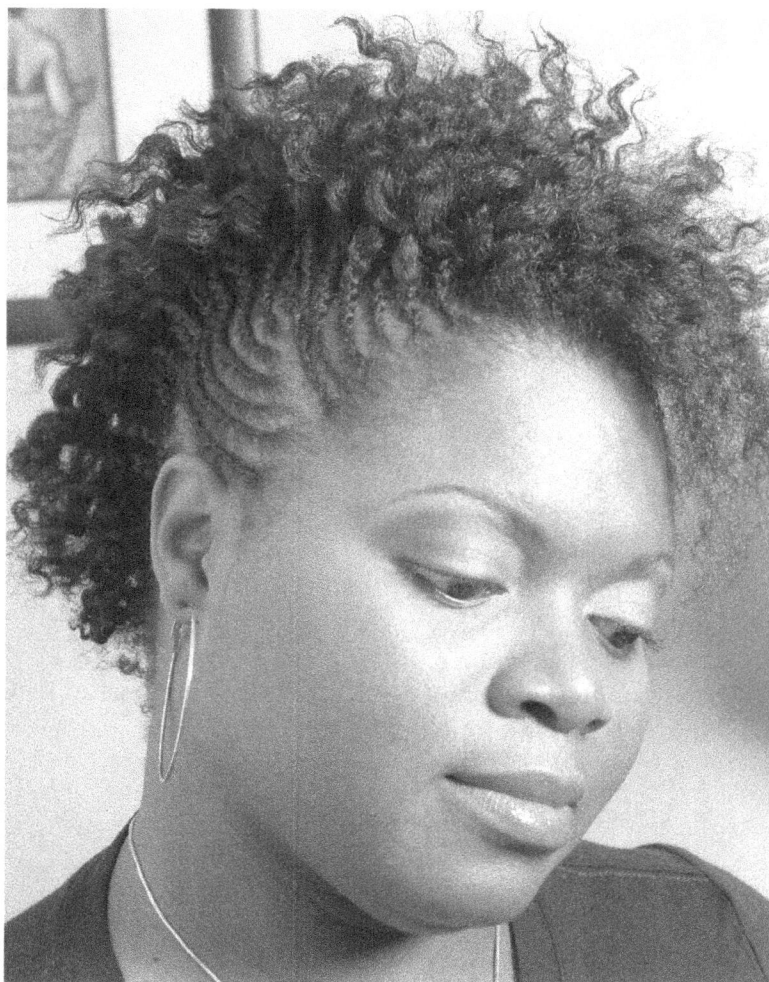

Hair: Simone Hylton, Natural Trendsetters, Makeup: Camille Belle. Photo: Justice Photography

This is Anna's twist outs using the Nairobi Wrapp Lotion, with the back flat-twisted upwards on a slant. Once again, she slept with the twists overnight. Her twist outs lasted all week as well:

With the twists: Finished results:

Hair: Simone Hylton, Natural Trendsetters, Makeup: Giselle Telesford. Photo: Justice Photography

This style she did herself – braiding the front half with bantu knots in the back. She then just inserted a decorative band for added flair:

Anna has been having alot of fun with her hair, and I am very excited! This is her recent twists that she did herself with the Taliah Waajid Lock it Up gel; they were very defined when she took them out and soft, and the twists were a beautiful style all by themselves:

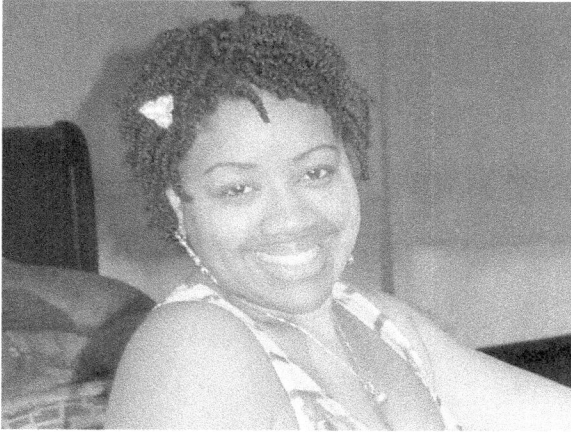

The longer her hair gets, the more she branches out and tries new things with it. This is the back view of her recent puff:

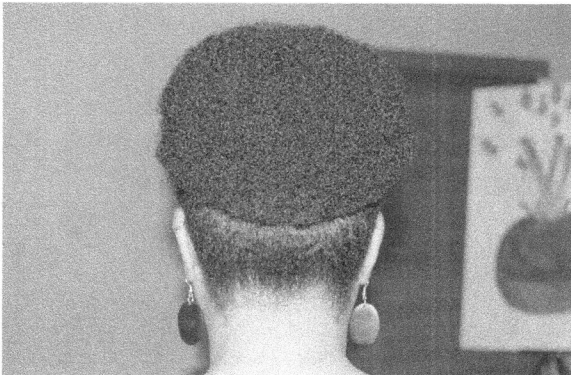

Sorry for the quality; these are from my cell phone. These big twists (I only had three on each side; had to do wet, or it wouldn't stay), gave me these size curls:

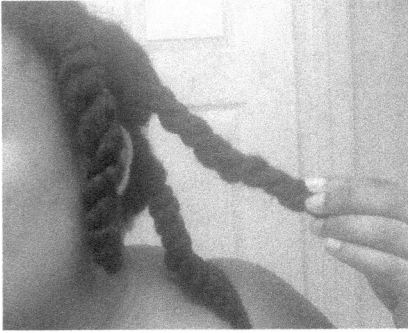

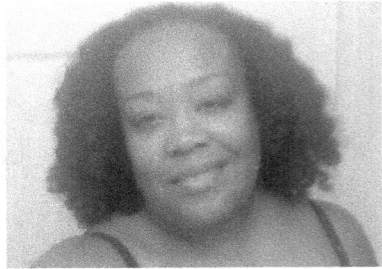

And these braids, when taken out, gave me these size waves:

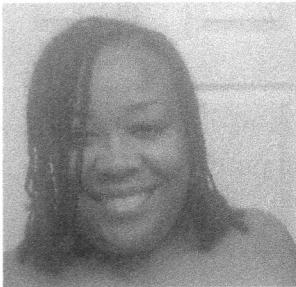

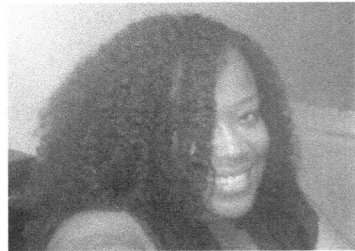

This is the normal size of twists I wear to achieve the look I use the most. Maybe 10-14 twists in all. I'd wear them all week to work, then wear the twist outs over the weekend. I love them:

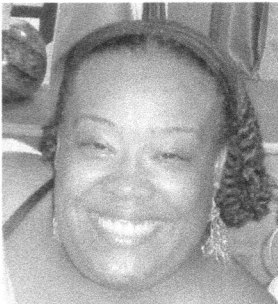

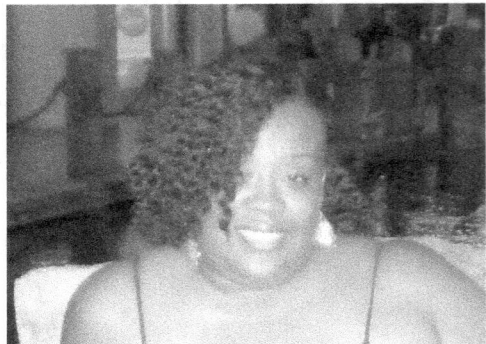

Stretching Out Your Curls

So after taking extra special care with your hair and it has grown so long, there's absolutely nothing wrong with wanting to show off more of your length. One way to do this when you're wearing your hair curly is to use a blow dryer on low heat and high speed, grab the bottom half of your hair by cupping the curls in your hands (to keep those curls and ends intact) and pull the roots out straight, while giving it a blast of air from the blow dryer. You'll want to do this on the underside of your hair as opposed to the top, so that the top of the hair still maintains the curly look from the roots. Let go, and grab another section. Repeat until you've completed the entire head. You should definitely see a considerable difference in length and volume, decreasing shrinkage.

Another way if you don't want to use heat is to braid your hair in Big Braids (four to six sections or so, depending on your length and the definition desired). After loosening the braids the next day, your hair will be stretched out more than your normal shrinkage pattern, and you will have loose waves.

Another method some use is simply wearing their hair in a bun (when you twist and wrap the hair around until it's all in a knot, like a Bantu Knot. The hair doesn't get a chance to shrink excessively, and when you take it out, it results in looser curls. This method, of course, is for longer hair.

Finally, yet another method is called banding. Banding is when you divide your hair into several sections and use several coated rubber bands on each section, banding the hair from the root all the way down to the tip, to keep the hair in a stretched-out condition. The spacing between the bands in each section varies, depending on how tight your curls are and how long your hair is. My only problem with banding is it leaves the sections in your hair sticking out straight, like branches on a tree. I don't know how people sleep like that, LOL, but it does work in stretching out your hair.

The longer your hair gets, the more you will want to stretch it out a bit when you're wearing it loose. Not just to show off more length, but also for manageability; when your hair is long, thick, and curly, it can be quite an experience to leave it out and wear it in a loose style. You can feel like hair is everywhere, and may end up (like I have on many occasions) pulling it back in a ponytail, just to get it under control. My hair is so curly and thick, something as small as giving someone a hug without having hair all in his or her face can be a challenge. Stretching out the curls with a twist, braid, or Bantu knot-out style can make the hair significantly more controllable, and easier to maintain a style all day or night.

Conclusion

Healthy, natural hair gives you so many options. The hair is thick, it grows, it's strong, it's curly, it's bouncy, and it's beautiful. You have so many options with your natural hair, and can straighten it whenever you want a change, while still maintaining your healthy hair. I hope that this book has given you some insight on a few things: the way you think about your own natural hair, how to take care of it, how to maintain length, and how to strengthen your locks.

I originally wanted to subtitle this book "How to embrace your natural hair," but I later realized that is something I cannot do for an individual. I do hope however, that the information you attained from this book will help you to do that on your own; because embracing what is yours and a part of you is a beautiful, enlightening, and freeing experience.

Please feel free to visit us at reclaimnaturalbeauty.com to share experiences, methods, products, styling tools and hairstyles; or maybe pick up some HOMEGROWN™ apparel for your stylish wardrobe.

Above all, please remember, REAL BEAUTY is HOMEGROWN™.

Bless.

****

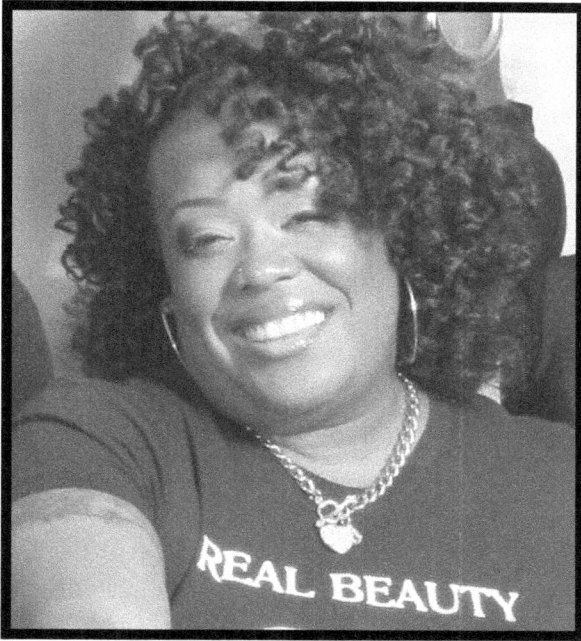

About the Author

Camille Jefferson was born and raised in Brooklyn, New York, and moved to Miami, Fl in 1999. She is a Writer, Editor and Graphic Designer, and lives in Florida with her two children.

www.ingramcontent.com/pod-product-compliance
Lightning Source LLC
Chambersburg PA
CBHW060855280326
41934CB00007B/1053